Department of Veterans Affairs
Health Services Research & Development Service | Evidence-based Synthesis Program

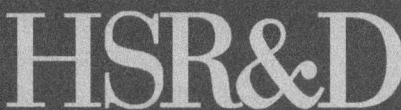

I0470877

The Effect of Working Conditions on Patient Care: A Systematic Review

January 2012

Prepared for:
Department of Veterans Affairs
Veterans Health Administration
Health Services Research & Development Service
Washington, DC 20420

Prepared by:
Evidence-based Synthesis Program (ESP) Center
Minneapolis VA Medical Center
Minneapolis, MN
Timothy J. Wilt, MD, MPH, Director

Investigators:
Principal Investigator:
Kandice A. Kapinos, PhD

Research Associates:
Patrick Fitzgerald, MPH
Nancy Greer, PhD
Indulis Rutks, BS

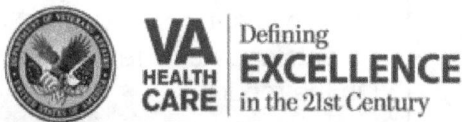

PREFACE

Health Services Research & Development Service's (HSR&D's) Evidence-based Synthesis Program (ESP) was established to provide timely and accurate syntheses of targeted healthcare topics of particular importance to Veterans Affairs (VA) managers and policymakers, as they work to improve the health and healthcare of Veterans. The ESP disseminates these reports throughout VA.

HSR&D provides funding for four ESP Centers and each Center has an active VA affiliation. The ESP Centers generate evidence syntheses on important clinical practice topics, and these reports help:

- develop clinical policies informed by evidence,
- guide the implementation of effective services to improve patient outcomes and to support VA clinical practice guidelines and performance measures, and
- set the direction for future research to address gaps in clinical knowledge.

In 2009, the ESP Coordinating Center was created to expand the capacity of HSR&D Central Office and the four ESP sites by developing and maintaining program processes. In addition, the Center established a Steering Committee comprised of HSR&D field-based investigators, VA Patient Care Services, Office of Quality and Performance, and Veterans Integrated Service Networks (VISN) Clinical Management Officers. The Steering Committee provides program oversight, guides strategic planning, coordinates dissemination activities, and develops collaborations with VA leadership to identify new ESP topics of importance to Veterans and the VA healthcare system.

Comments on this evidence report are welcome and can be sent to Nicole Floyd, ESP Coordinating Center Program Manager, at nicole.floyd@va.gov.

Recommended citation: Kapinos KA, Fitzgerald P, Greer N, Rutks I, Wilt TJ. The Effect of Working Conditions on Patient Care: A Systematic Review. VA-ESP Project #09-009; 2012.

This report is based on research conducted by the Evidence-based Synthesis Program (ESP) Center located at the Minneapolis VA Medical Center, Minneapolis, MN funded by the Department of Veterans Affairs, Veterans Health Administration, Office of Research and Development, Health Services Research and Development. The findings and conclusions in this document are those of the author(s) who are responsible for its contents; the findings and conclusions do not necessarily represent the views of the Department of Veterans Affairs or the United States government. Therefore, no statement in this article should be construed as an official position of the Department of Veterans Affairs. No investigators have any affiliations or financial involvement (e.g., employment, consultancies, honoraria, stock ownership or options, expert testimony, grants or patents received or pending, or royalties) that conflict with material presented in the report.

TABLE OF CONTENTS

EXECUTIVE SUMMARY

Background 1

Methods 1

Data Synthesis 2

Peer Review 2

Results 2

Conclusions 4

Future Research 5

INTRODUCTION

Background 6

Working Conditions 7

Conceptual Model 8

Patient Outcomes 9

Provider Outcomes 10

METHODS

Topic Development 12

Search Strategy 13

Study Selection 13

Data Abstraction 13

Quality Assessment 13

Data Synthesis 14

Rating the Body of Evidence 14

Peer Review 14

RESULTS

Literature Flow 15

Key Question #1. How are human resources (HR) practices, such as skill levels, training,
workload, hours worked, autonomy, and electronic medical records/systems, associated
with patient outcomes? 17

Key Question #2. How are other working conditions, such as organizational culture or physical
environment, associated with patient outcomes? 24

Key Question #3. In studies that report provider outcomes, how are working conditions
associated with provider outcomes (e.g., job satisfaction, productivity, pay)? 30

SUMMARY AND DISCUSSION

Summary of Evidence by Key Question 32

Recommendations for Future Research 34

Conclusions 34

REFERENCES 36

TABLES

Table 1.　Human Resource Practices Studies by HR Practice Studied and Patient Outcome Studied..... 18

Table 2.　Human Resource Practices – Strength of Evidence for Key Outcomes................................... 24

Table 3.　Organizational Culture Studies by Practice Studied and Patient Outcome Studied................. 26

Table 4.　Physical Environment Studies by Patient Outcome Studied.. 28

Table 5.　Physical Environment Outcomes 29

FIGURES

Figure 1.　Conceptual Model – Quality of Care in Primary Care.. 9

Figure 2.　Analytic Framework... 12

Figure 3.　Literature Flow Diagram – Human Resource Practices Studies 15

Figure 4.　Literature Flow Diagram – Organizational Culture Studies.. 16

Figure 5.　Literature Flow Diagram – Physical Environment Studies.. 16

Figure 6.　Study Quality of Human Resource Practices Non-Randomized Studies 23

Figure 7.　Study Quality of Organizational Culture Non-Randomized Studies...................................... 28

Figure 8.　Study Quality of Physical Environment Non-Randomized Studies.. 30

APPENDIX A. SEARCH STRATEGIES 42

APPENDIX B. CRITERIA USED IN QUALITY ASSESSMENT OF NON-RANDOMIZED STUDIES............. 44

APPENDIX C. PEER REVIEW COMMENTS/AUTHOR RESPONSES.. 45

APPENDIX D. EVIDENCE TABLES

Table 1.　Description of Human Resources Practices Studies – United States 48

Table 2.　Description of Human Resources Practices Studies – Europe 51

Table 3.　Description of Human Resources Practices Studies – Outside of US or Europe...................... 53

Table 4.　Quality of Care Outcomes – Human Resource Practices Studies 54

Table 5.　Patient Safety Outcomes – Human Resource Practices Studies... 56

Table 6.　Patient Satisfaction Outcomes – Human Resource Practices Studies 57

Table 7.　Description of Organizational Culture Studies.. 59

Table 8.　Quality of Care Outcomes – Organizational Culture Studies... 63

Table 9.　Patient Safety Outcomes – Organizational Culture Studies 64

Table 10.　Patient Satisfaction Outcomes – Organizational Culture Studies 65

Table 11.　Provider Outcomes – Organizational Culture Studies... 66

Table 12.　Description of Physical Environment Studies... 67

EXECUTIVE SUMMARY

BACKGROUND

A large body of evidence shows clear linkages between workplace conditions and employee satisfaction and stress in a wide variety of organizational and industry settings. In the healthcare industry, increasing interest in understanding these linkages stems from the idea that healthcare providers' working environments also affect important patient outcomes, including safety, quality of care and satisfaction. Additionally, meeting objectives of the current healthcare reform to increase healthcare quality by increasing the availability of primary care providers and making care safer, more efficient, effective and patient-centered hinges on the ability to deal with the documented shortage of primary care providers in the US and at the same time improve patient outcomes. The purpose of this report was to systematically review the evidence on the role of primary care providers' workplace conditions in influencing patient outcomes. We focused on patient satisfaction, safety, and quality of care for patient outcomes (note that there may be some overlap in how these patient outcomes are measured). We excluded articles that focused on one specific disease or patient population. The focus on primary care providers' work environment will provide evidence on increasing healthcare quality. Results from this review may inform policymakers as they endeavor to implement aspects of the healthcare reform related to increasing the supply of primary care providers and improving patient outcomes.

The key questions were:

Key Question #1. How are human resources (HR) practices, such as skill levels, training, workload, hours worked, autonomy, and electronic medical records/systems, associated with patient outcomes?

>   a. quality of care (access and effectiveness)
>   b. safety (medication errors)
>   c. patient satisfaction (with provider, with clinic/practice)

Key Question #2. How are other working conditions, such as organizational culture or physical environment, associated with patient outcomes?

>   a. quality of care (access and effectiveness)
>   b. safety (medication errors)
>   c. patient satisfaction (with provider, with clinic/practice)

Key Question #3. In studies that report provider outcomes, how are working conditions associated with provider outcomes (e.g., job satisfaction, productivity, pay)?

METHODS

We conducted searches for each of the workplace conditions (i.e., human resource practices [separate searches for staffing and workflow], organizational culture, and physical environment) in MEDLINE and PsycINFO using standard search terms. We also searched both MEDLINE and PsycINFO for studies of team-based approaches to care. We included randomized controlled trials (RCTs), systematic reviews, and prospective studies published in English from 2000 to September 2011. Our search focused on primary care physicians, nurse practitioners, and physician assistants as providers and adult patients. For provider outcomes, we searched MEDLINE and the Cochrane Effective Practice and Organization of Care (EPOC) Group Web site for recent systematic reviews or meta-analyses. We excluded articles that focused on one disease or patient population (e.g., diabetes or depression), lacked data analysis, or focused on the effect of credentials or skills (i.e., MD [physician] vs. PA [physician assistant] or NP [nurse practitioner]) on quality of care or patient safety. We excluded the latter studies as there is already a body of evidence suggesting that increased skills improve clinical effectiveness (see Agency for Healthcare Research and Quality [AHRQ] report 2003). All searches were limited to articles pertaining to human subjects and published in the English language. Additional citations were identified from reference lists of related articles.

Titles, abstracts, and articles were reviewed by researchers trained in critical analysis of literature. We attempted to pool data if appropriate. Other data were summarized narratively.

Study characteristics, patient characteristics, and outcomes were extracted by a trained research associate under the supervision of the Principal Investigator. We assessed risk of bias in individual studies according to established criteria for randomized controlled trials and based on population, outcomes, measurement, and confounding for non-randomized trials. Strength of evidence was determined for primary outcomes.

DATA SYNTHESIS

We constructed evidence tables for study characteristics and for outcomes, organized by working condition. We analyzed studies to compare their characteristics, methods, and findings. Findings from VA or active service populations were identified and highlighted.

PEER REVIEW

A draft version of this report was reviewed by members of our technical expert panel, as well as clinical leadership. Reviewer comments were addressed and our responses were incorporated in the final report (Appendix C).

RESULTS

The Effect of Human Resources Practices (Key Question #1)

For Key Question #1, we screened 1008 abstracts and 95 full text articles related to staffing and 1,581 abstracts and 94 full text articles related to workflow. We included 14 references from the staffing search and 9 references from the workflow search. Four additional references were added from our hand search of reference lists for a total of 27 references. Among these studies, three were randomized controlled trials, seven were longitudinal (cohort or pre-post with repeated cross-sections) studies and 17 were cross-sectional.

Nine out of eleven of the studies we examined that focused on patient quality of care as an outcome specifically measured clinical effectiveness, thus there is insufficient evidence on the role of provider workplace conditions on access as a quality of care measure. The most frequently studied HR practice for quality of care was workload and while three of the studies suggested that an increase in workload results in lower quality of care, one study also found a positive effect and one found no effect. The other HR practices studied were evaluated less frequently, but there was more consistency in the results across studies: more training (2 studies), shorter hours (2 studies), and computerized systems (3 studies) lead to better quality. Only one study we reviewed examined provider autonomy or flexibility and found mixed effects on quality of care scores; this is insufficient evidence for the role of autonomy. Overall, these results are suggestive but make it difficult to make strong conclusions about the role of HR practices on patient quality of care.

We identified four studies in our review that explicitly examined the role of workplace conditions on patient safety in the primary care setting. While these were relatively well designed studies, more studies are needed. Because only two studies examined workload, one examined autonomy, one examined teams, and one examined computerized systems, there is insufficient evidence to answer our key question about how HR practices influence patient safety.

We identified 17 unique studies that investigated how HR practices influence patient satisfaction with either the provider or the clinic. We found mixed evidence on the role of provider skills (MD vs. NP/PA) on patient satisfaction; two studies found no effect and two studies found a negative effect of skills. We found mostly no effect of provider workload on patient satisfaction (3 studies), with the exception of one Norwegian study reporting that a longer listsize resulted in greater patient satisfaction. All four of the studies that examined provider training and all three that examined provider work hours found that they had no effect on patient satisfaction. Thus, there was suggestive evidence that training and work hours do not effect patient satisfaction, but again because of the lack of well-designed studies, we cannot make strong conclusions about these findings. Similarly, we conclude that there is inconsistent evidence on the role of skills and workload. We identified no studies that looked at how electronic medical records or computerized systems affect patient satisfaction.

The Effect of Organizational Culture and Physical Environment (Key Question #2)

For Key Question #2, we screened 541 abstracts and 44 full text references from our search for studies related to organizational culture. We included 2 references from our organizational culture literature search, 1 reference from our team-based care literature search, and 6 references that were identified by hand searching. Our physical environment search yielded 49 abstracts to review. From the 49 abstracts, we reviewed 3 full text articles; none met inclusion criteria. We included 2 references identified by hand searching.

Our findings on the effect of organizational culture are similar to findings of earlier reviews. The diversity of study methodologies used and constructs of organizational culture studied and the lack of consistent and validated outcome measures limit the ability to draw conclusions. Two studies (one randomized controlled trial and one pre/post study) found a positive effect of provider teams on patient quality of care, though one found no effect (case control study). Two studies that examined the effect of implementing patient centered medical homes (PCMH) found positive effects on quality of care. A cross-sectional study also found that organizations with an organizational culture that emphasized the importance of information sharing had high quality of care.

Although there has been research on the effect of physical environment (notably lighting, color, auditory stimuli, and temperature) on workplace performance, much of that work has been done in industrial settings and what has been done in healthcare has largely focused on hospitals rather than the primary care setting.

Provider Outcomes (Key Question #3)

For Key Question #3, we included provider outcomes from studies identified in the literature searches for Key Questions #1 and #2. We also included systematic reviews pertaining to provider outcomes in primary care.

The relationships between workplace conditions, provider outcomes, and patient outcomes are complex and dynamic in such a way that not only are the effects felt at many levels (provider, patient, healthcare system), but also they create a cycle of reinforcing behaviors and outcomes. There are several potential policy interventions at the various levels that might positively influence provider well-being. In this study, we focused on studies that shed light on possible workplace interventions (as opposed to provider self-care or higher-order system level interventions) that could ultimately impact patient outcomes. Such changes to workplace conditions will likely also influence provider outcomes. However, we presented these results as only suggestive, but consistent with other literature, that has established evidence on the intermediate link between workplace conditions and provider outcomes.

Strength of Evidence

We evaluated the strength of evidence for the workplace conditions and patient outcomes for which we had at least three studies. Strength of evidence overall was low for patient satisfaction and provider skills, workload and hours; and for quality of care and provider workload and electronic medical records. Most of the evidence was rated high or moderate on risk of bias due to the lack of many well-designed RCTs or observational studies that address potential biases. There was also inconsistent measurement of both the workplace condition constructs and the patient outcome constructs, which made comparisons across studies difficult. There was insufficient evidence for patient safety and all workplace conditions, quality of care and training and hours, and patient satisfaction and electronic medical records (EMRs). Additionally, there was insufficient evidence on provider autonomy and all patient outcomes.

CONCLUSIONS

Overall, the studies we reviewed suggest that in primary care settings

- a lighter provider workload/shorter work hours, more provider training, and computerized systems result in higher patient quality of care
- provider training and work hours have no effect on patient satisfaction.

We found mixed evidence on the effect of provider skill levels and workload on patient satisfaction. We identified very few studies in our review that explicitly examined the role of workplace conditions on patient safety or the role of the physical environment on patient outcomes in the primary care setting, thus more studies are needed. Several workplace conditions have been insufficiently studied and thus there is no evidence on how these practices matter in ambulatory care settings: the effect of computerized systems, provider autonomy and teams on patient satisfaction; the effect of autonomy on quality of care.

The available literature provides low strength or insufficient evidence for varied components of organizational culture including PCMH, team-based care, care environment, and clinic values and their effect on outcomes highlighted in our key questions. Such evidence does not permit conclusions with regard to quality of care, patient safety, and patient satisfaction.

We found two studies that focused on the effect of physical environment in primary care clinics. No study attempted to isolate any one component of the physical environment. Reported outcomes included self-report of satisfaction (worker and provider/staff) with no objective measures of patient safety or quality of care or provider performance.

Consistent with more thorough systematic reviews of the literature examining how workplace conditions affect providers' stress, job satisfaction, etc., among the studies in our review that also examined provider outcomes, we found that greater workloads and less control over work tasks resulted in greater provider stress, burnout, and less job satisfaction. One study we examined found that electronic medical records did not result in greater provider stress.

FUTURE RESEARCH

There is little research that investigates the effects of working conditions on patient safety, which we measure specifically as medication errors, in the primary care setting. More generally, more well-designed studies are needed to replicate the few that have been conducted. For example, all ten of the studies we reviewed that investigated the role of workload were cross-sectional studies. While undertaking randomized controlled trials may be impractical, well-designed cohort studies or other pre-post designs will allow for more convincing evidence on the causal effect of the workplace conditions. Additionally, there is a need for research that looks rigorously at the interdependent role of human resource practices (such as hours worked, provider autonomy, and electronic medical records), organizational culture, and physical environment in explaining patient outcomes in primary care settings. For example, implementation of team-based work is often accompanied by other changes in the workplace, such as the use of electronic medical records/computerized systems or changes in organizational culture to foster teamwork. Therefore, any changes in patient outcomes from such an implementation could be the result of the teamwork, but could also be attributable to the changes in the organizational culture or computerized systems, etc. Current studies do not adequately try to isolate these effects. Finally, the development of or more consistent use of construct valid measures of both working conditions and patient or provider outcomes in the primary care settings is needed to make comparisons across studies easier.

EVIDENCE REPORT

INTRODUCTION

A patient safety movement that began with a 1999 Institute of Medicine report on the prevalence of preventable medical errors has spawned both policy to change health care systems and a growing body of literature aimed at understanding the causes of such errors.[1-3] A 2003 AHRQ systematic review investigated the role that workplace conditions play in explaining patient safety and found that workloads, work schedules, lengths of work shifts, and stress levels affected rates of non-fatal adverse outcomes, mortality rates, medication errors, and other patient safety measures.[4] However, much of this evidence relies on studies based in hospitals and focuses on nurse and resident staffing or is based on studies in non-healthcare settings.

BACKGROUND

A large body of evidence has shown clear linkages between workplace conditions and employee satisfaction and stress in a wide variety of organizational and industry settings.[5] In the healthcare industry, increasing interest in understanding these linkages has stemmed from the idea that healthcare providers' working environments also affect important patient outcomes, including safety, quality of care and satisfaction.[6] Additionally, meeting objectives of the current healthcare reform to increase healthcare quality by increasing the availability of primary care providers and making care safer, more efficient, effective and patient-centered hinges on the ability to deal with the documented shortage of primary care providers in the US[7,8] and at the same time improve patient outcomes.

The purpose of this report is to systematically review the evidence on the role of primary care providers' workplace conditions in influencing patient outcomes. The focus on primary care providers' work environment will provide evidence on increasing healthcare quality. While the focus of this review is on patient outcomes, we do discuss implications for providers and recent review studies that highlight the importance of provider wellness as a component of high quality care.[9] Results from this review may inform policymakers as they endeavor to implement aspects of the healthcare reform related to increasing the supply of primary care providers and improving patient outcomes.

Following the 2003 AHRQ report,[4] we focused on the following workplace conditions: 1) human resource practices 2) organizational culture, and 3) physical environment, but restricted our review to studies on primary care providers (physicians, physician assistants, and nurse practitioners) in ambulatory care settings. Note that the workplace condition constructs, specifically "human resources practices" and "organizational culture", may overlap. However, our categorization of these workplace conditions does not affect the evidence presented; it merely serves as a way to organize a long list of workplace conditions. As mentioned above, we restricted our analysis to studies focused on the following patient outcomes, broadly defined: patient care quality, medical errors, patient safety, and patient satisfaction. We conceptualized primary or ambulatory care to include clinics and providers that serve as a first point of contact for patients where common illnesses and conditions are treated. Therefore, we excluded studies that focused on one specific disease, even chronic conditions that may be managed by a primary care provider, or one specific patient population (e.g. diabetics). We discuss these work environment concepts, patient safety measures, and our conceptual model below.

WORKING CONDITIONS

Our key questions, study protocol and populations, interventions, settings and outcomes of interest were guided by consultation with a panel of experts.

We delineated workplace conditions of primary care providers into three categories: human resources practices, organizational culture and physical environment. Note that some elements of "human resources practices" could conceivably be classified as characteristics of a workplace's organizational culture (and vice versa), but we have roughly followed the categorizations from the 2003 AHRQ report.[4] In another AHRQ report,[10] the authors describe elements of organizational climate as part of the healthcare structures, whereas the actual workplace practices are part of the processes (see also our conceptual model below). These workplace condition classifications are simply geared at organizing the presentation of results and do not change or in any way shape the evidence presented. Note that many of these constructs are measured in varied ways across studies. We mention some of the most commonly used measures below and provide details on the measures used in each study in Appendix D, Tables 1-3, 7, and 12.

Human Resources Practices

Human resources practices encompass all organizational practices and policies that pertain to managing employees. In this study, we focused on skill levels/training and work systems. Skill levels and training reflect some measure of knowledge, either through formal general training (i.e., physician vs. nurse practitioner) or more specific training aimed at increasing providers' knowledge or skills in helping patients. Note that we did not include studies that investigated the effect of disease specific training on patient outcomes. Work systems include workload, scheduling, autonomy, and other systems or structures in place that affect how providers do their jobs, such as electronic medical records or computerized systems. Workload is typically measured as the "listsize" (number of patients a physician has), by the number of procedures performed, the number of patients seen, and time pressures related to work pace. A related concept is provider scheduling, which may be measured as shift length, typical hours, or days of the week worked. Scheduling is studied less in the ambulatory care setting than in the hospital setting. Autonomy or control of one's work refers to the flexibility that providers have in exactly how they get their tasks completed.

While pay systems, and in particular pay for performance settings, are an important component of workplace conditions and human resource practices that likely influence patient (and provider) outcomes, we do not systematically review this literature in this report. There is a large existing literature on pay for performance spanning several disciplines, in general, but also a large growing literature on this topic in healthcare settings. We discuss recent systematic reviews on this topic below.

Organizational Culture

Organizational culture pertains to issues related to the social norms in a workplace. We focused on studies that investigated organizational climate, professional culture, and the structural organization or hierarchies present in a workplace, including the use of teams. Organizational climate includes provider perceptions of how open the organization is to change, what is valued at the organization (e.g. patient safety, learning), and expectations about how to work and fit in at the organization. For example, one VA study identified the following factors of organizational climate: employee focus, support (group processes and supervision), and professional demands.[11] Professional culture involves how value perceptions vary across different professions within the organization and how teamwork and relationships within the organization are valued. Finally, in this study, organizational culture encompasses organizational structures or hierarchies related to the division of labor within an organization. We include "team-based care" as a component of organizational culture as it is often accompanied with other cultural or structural characteristics that facilitate teamwork. The literature on healthcare teams (and related concepts such as patient centered care) is large, but for this review, we focused on studies that investigated the effectiveness of teams where at least one team member is a physician, nurse practitioner, or physician assistant.

Physical Environment

Physical environment pertains to issues related to the direct physical characteristics of the workplace. We focused on studies that investigate environmental safety, lighting, temperature, and physical layout of clinics. Environmental safety includes air quality, indoor pollution, toxic exposures, and noise. The physical environment also includes aesthetic and comfort aspects of the workplace, such as lighting, temperature, and humidity. Finally, the physical layout at the workplace, such as whether there are obstacles or large distances between work stations, may influence patient outcomes.

CONCEPTUAL MODEL

We draw from several quality of care models from the nurse staffing literature that build on Donabedian's work delineating quality as it relates to healthcare structures, processes, and outcomes.[12] In Figure 1, we outline the main model noting that these relationships can also be outlined at different levels, including individual, group, organizational or system. We also note that this model can easily be expanded with the complexity added due to interactions at various levels and the possibility of bidirectional effects (of say, structures and processes).[13] Additionally, we have included intermediary outcomes in this model; in particular, we highlight that an underlying behavioral mechanism exists whereby the organizational structures and processes affect provider's job satisfaction, productivity, pay, and similar outcomes. Studies that focused solely on these intermediary outcomes are beyond the scope of this report. For the purposes of this report, we focused on the general effect of workplace conditions and related clinical processes on patient outcomes.

Figure 1. Conceptual Model – Quality of Care in Primary Care

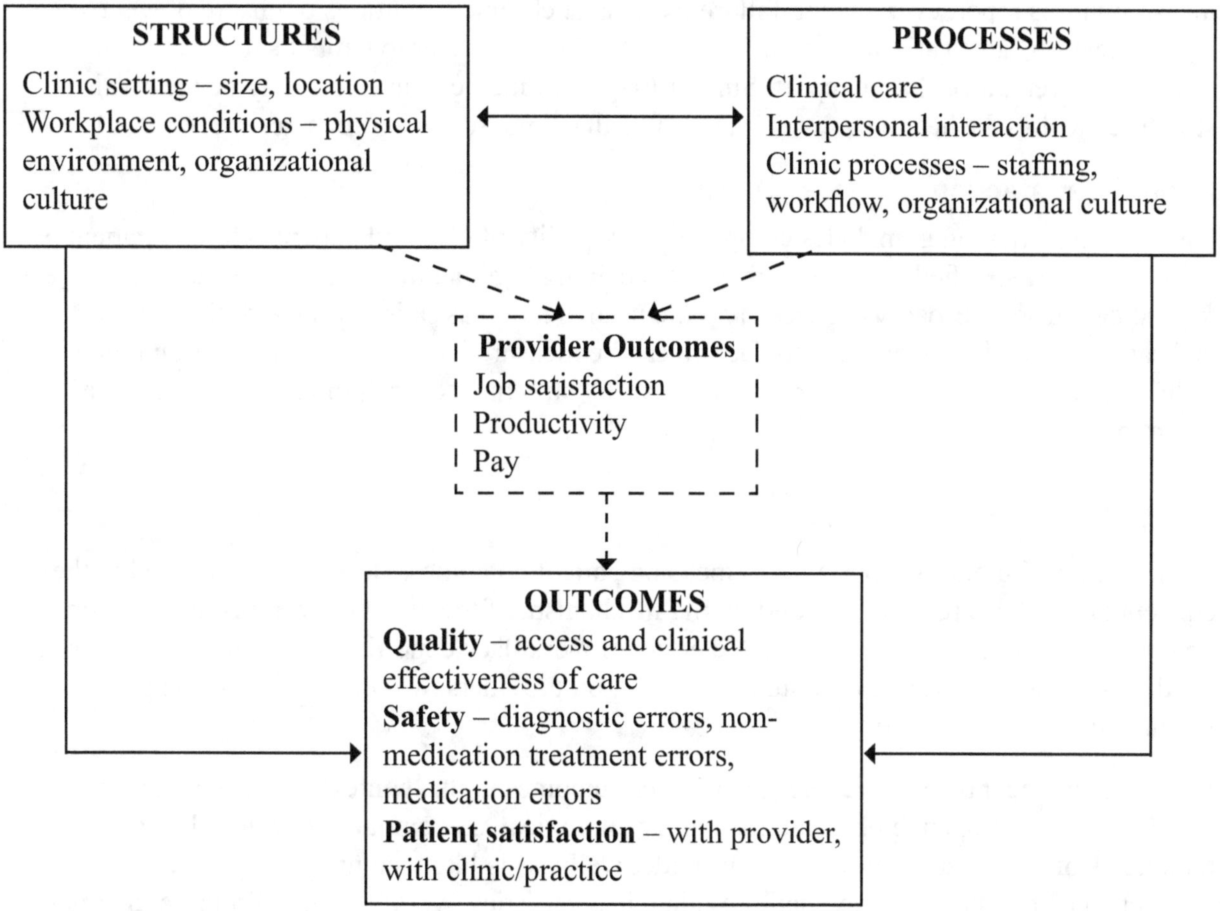

```
┌─────────────────────────────────────┐          ┌─────────────────────────────────────┐
│           STRUCTURES                 │          │           PROCESSES                 │
│  Clinic setting – size, location     │ ◄──────► │  Clinical care                      │
│  Workplace conditions – physical     │          │  Interpersonal interaction          │
│  environment, organizational         │          │  Clinic processes – staffing,       │
│  culture                             │          │  workflow, organizational culture   │
└─────────────────────────────────────┘          └─────────────────────────────────────┘
```

┌ ─ ─ ─ ─ ─ ─ ─ ─ ─ ─ ─ ┐
│ **Provider Outcomes** │
│ Job satisfaction   │
│ Productivity   │
│ Pay   │
└ ─ ─ ─ ─ ─ ─ ─ ─ ─ ─ ─ ┘

```
┌─────────────────────────────────────┐
│              OUTCOMES                │
│  **Quality** – access and clinical  │
│  effectiveness of care              │
│  **Safety** – diagnostic errors, non-│
│  medication treatment errors,       │
│  medication errors                  │
│  **Patient satisfaction** – with provider,│
│  with clinic/practice               │
└─────────────────────────────────────┘
```

PATIENT OUTCOMES

We focused on the following patient outcomes: quality of care, patient safety, and patient satisfaction.

Quality of Care

Quality of care is typically categorized broadly into a)access to care and b)effectiveness of care.[14] Accessibility addresses whether patients can actually get the care they need while clinical effectiveness addresses whether the care received results in the intended outcome. Both constructs are influenced by structures and processes in the healthcare setting. For example, access can be limited by both physical location (structure) and affordability (process). Effectiveness includes knowledge or evidence-based care, guideline concordant care, or clinical effectiveness and is often measured as provider compliance to the guidelines or evidence.

Patient Safety

Patient safety can be broadly related to diagnosis errors, treatment errors, and perhaps missing preventive services.[15] However, because there is some overlap in treatment and diagnostic errors with quality of care, we included performance metrics dealing with missing preventive services or other metrics that represent management of disease or appropriate care with the quality measure in this report even though failure to manage chronic conditions or ensure preventive care utilization can clearly lead to adverse events. Thus, we refer to patient safety as medication errors in the remainder of the report. Similar to quality, medication errors may be the result of structures within the health care system or clinical and non-clinical processes.

Patient Satisfaction

Patient satisfaction often includes components of quality of care and patient safety as patients tend to be more satisfied if they feel they are receiving high quality care and they are not subject to medical errors.[16] Broadly, we classify patient satisfaction as satisfaction with the provider and satisfaction with the clinic. Satisfaction can be measured using different scales and may be influenced as much by clinical care processes as by structures or the clinic environment (i.e., receptionist, waiting time, etc.).

PROVIDER OUTCOMES

As noted, the aim of this report was to focus on patient outcomes. However, as outlined in the conceptual model (Figure 1), the underlying mechanism of the effect of workplace conditions on patient outcomes is likely through the effect of workplace conditions on *providers*. Although we did not systematically review studies focused on providers, we briefly discuss the general findings from this literature.

Following a recent review, we refer to provider outcomes in this context as aspects of provider "wellness," which include physical, mental/psychological, and emotional health.[9] Understanding the effects of workplace conditions on provider wellness is likely complicated by the interdependent nature the individual provider characteristics, workplace conditions, and larger healthcare system factors.

One of the most frequently studied provider outcomes is psychological stress, which correlates with poor physical and mental health. Various healthcare workplace conditions have been linked to increased stress levels and negative physical health for providers, including workload, pay, organizational structure (bureaucratic), restricted autonomy, and a professional culture that does not encourage providers to seek medical help for themselves.[9]

Beyond the immediate physical and mental health effects of workplace conditions on providers are the effects that ripple through the healthcare system. The effects of job stress on healthcare providers' absenteeism, burnout, performance, and intention to quit or leave,[17-20] have been well documented in the literature. Not surprisingly, stressed employees are more likely to be absent from work, be low performers, and have greater turnover rates than other employees. Similarly, satisfied providers are more likely to have satisfied patients.[21,22] At the organizational level, these effects can permeate the organizational culture to create an unhealthy and ineffective workforce.[20,23] Furthermore, stressed and dissatisfied healthcare providers are more likely to make medical mistakes that effect patients[24-26] and have dissatisfied patients.[27]

As noted above, these relationships are complex and dynamic in such a way that not only are the effects felt at many levels (provider, patient, healthcare system), but also they create a cycle of reinforcing behaviors and outcomes. For example, a heavy workload may cause a provider excessive psychological stress, which may in turn influence her physical health and also cause her to be more prone to medical errors, which may create even more distress repeating the cycle.[28,29]

As outlined in the Wallace et al. review,[9] there are several potential policy interventions at various levels that might positively influence provider wellbeing. In this study, we focused on studies that shed light on possible workplace interventions (as opposed to provider self-care or higher-order system level interventions) that will ultimately impact patient outcomes. Such changes to workplace conditions will likely <u>also</u> influence provider outcomes. While examples of workplace changes that positively affect both providers and patients exist, such as an organizational culture that emphasizes quality, reduces provider stress and increases quality of care for patients,[6] we point out that there are some workplace changes that may yield greater patient outcomes at the expense of poorer provider outcomes, such as electronic medical records.

METHODS

TOPIC DEVELOPMENT

This project was nominated by Michael Hodgson, MD, MPH. The primary aim was to review the evidence on the associations between primary care workplace conditions and patient outcomes as depicted in Figure 2. The key questions and scope of the report were refined with input from a technical expert panel.

The final key questions are:

Key Question #1. How are HR practices, such as skill levels, training, workload, hours worked, autonomy, and electronic medical records/systems, associated with patient outcomes?

    a. quality of care (access and effectiveness)
    b. safety (medication errors)
    c. patient satisfaction (with provider, with clinic/practice)

Key Question #2. How are other working conditions, such as organizational culture or physical environment, associated with patient outcomes?

    a. quality of care (access and effectiveness)
    b. safety (medication errors)
    c. patient satisfaction (with provider, with clinic/practice)

Key Question #3. In studies that report provider outcomes, how are HR practices and working conditions associated with provider outcomes (e.g., job satisfaction, productivity, pay)?

Figure 2. Analytic Framework

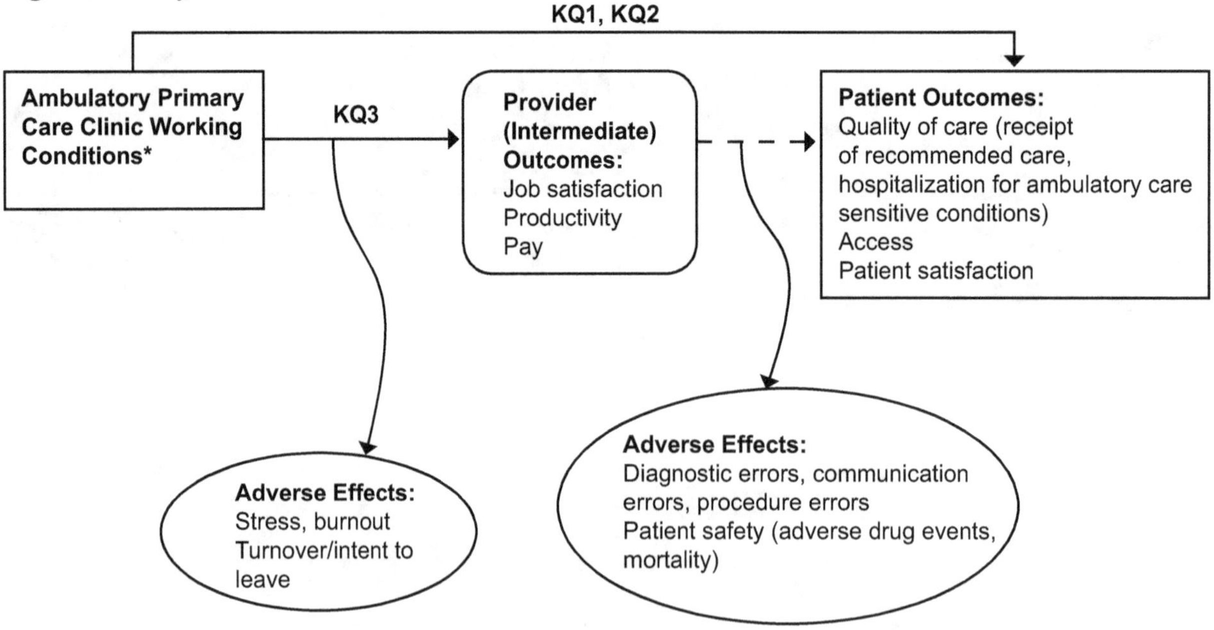

*Working Conditions of Ambulatory Primary Care Clinics
1. Human resources practices (work volume, scheduling, training/skills required, task design, information systems)
2. Organizational culture (organizational climate, professional culture, hierarchy)
3. Physical environment (safety, lighting/temperature, physical layout)

SEARCH STRATEGY

We conducted searches for human resource practices [separate searches for staffing and workflow], organizational culture, and physical environment in MEDLINE and PsycINFO. We developed our search strategies based on the 2003 AHRQ report.[4] To insure that we captured studies of team-based approaches to care (as requested by our TEP), we also did focused searches in both MEDLINE and PsycINFO. MEDLINE search strategies are presented in Appendix A. We included randomized controlled trials, systematic reviews, and prospective studies published in English from 2000 to September 2011. Our search focused on primary care physicians, nurse practitioners, and physician assistants as providers and adult patients receiving care in ambulatory, primary care settings. For provider outcomes, we searched MEDLINE and the Cochrane Effective Practice and Organization of Care (EPOC) Group Web site for recent systematic reviews or meta-analyses. Additional citations were identified from reference lists of related articles.

STUDY SELECTION

Titles and abstracts were reviewed by researchers trained in the critical analysis of literature. Full text versions of potentially eligible articles were retrieved for review. Our inclusion criteria were:

1. Study published in English language
2. Randomized trial, observational study or systematic review (the article had to present data analysis results)
3. Outpatient, adult, primary care setting, without focus on one specific disease or patient population
4. Study addressed working conditions for primary care physician, nurse practitioner, or physician assistant
5. Reported outcomes of interest:
   > Patient Outcomes – quality of care, patient safety, patient satisfaction
   > Provider Outcomes – job satisfaction, productivity, pay

DATA ABSTRACTION

We abstracted the following data for each included study for Key Questions #1 and #2: author, date of publication, country where study was conducted, funding source, characteristics of included patients, providers and/or clinics, study design, working conditions evaluated, and patient outcomes (quality [access, effectiveness], safety [medication errors], and satisfaction [with provider, with practice or care]). We also abstracted data on provider outcomes, where provided. Additional data for Key Question #3 was obtained from recent systematic reviews or meta-analyses. All abstraction was done by trained research personnel under the supervision of the Principal Investigator.

QUALITY ASSESSMENT

We assessed study quality of randomized trials according to the following criteria: 1) adequate allocation concealment, 2) blinding of key study personnel, 3) analysis by intention-to-treat, and 4) reporting of number of withdrawals/dropouts by group assignment.[30] Studies were rated as good, fair, or poor quality. A rating of good generally indicated that the trial reported adequate allocation concealment, appropriate blinding, analysis by intent-to-treat, and reasons for dropouts/attrition. Studies were generally rated poor if the method of allocation concealment was inadequate or not defined, blinding was not defined, analysis by intent-to-treat was not utilized, and reasons for dropouts/attrition were not reported and/or there was a high rate of attrition. For non-randomized trials, we determined risk of bias based on critical elements related to the population, intervention, outcomes, measurement, and confounding (Appendix B).

DATA SYNTHESIS

We constructed evidence tables showing the study characteristics and results for all included studies, organized by working condition. We critically analyzed studies to compare their characteristics, methods, and findings. Due to heterogeneity of interventions and outcomes assessed we were unable to pool results from different studies. We compiled a summary of findings for each working condition, and drew conclusions based on qualitative synthesis of the findings.

RATING THE BODY OF EVIDENCE

We assessed the overall quality of evidence using the method reported by Owens et al.[31] Briefly, for each outcome evaluated, the strength of the evidence was assessed based on: 1) risk of bias; 2) consistency; 3) directness; and 4) precision. Based on these four domains, the overall evidence was rated as: 1) high, meaning high confidence that the evidence reflects the true effect; 2) moderate, indicating moderate confidence that further research may change our confidence in the estimate of effect and may change the estimate; 3) low, meaning there is low confidence that the evidence reflects the true effect; and 4) insufficient, indicating that evidence either is unavailable or does not permit a conclusion.

PEER REVIEW

A draft version of this report was reviewed by members of our technical expert panel as well as VA clinical leadership. Their comments and our responses are presented in Appendix C.

RESULTS

LITERATURE FLOW

Figures 3-5 detail the exclusion criteria and the number of references related to each of the key questions. Separate searches were conducted for the human resource practices components of staffing and work flow. For the staffing search, we identified 1008 abstracts and excluded 913. Of 95 full text articles reviewed, we included 14. For the work flow search, we identified 1,581 abstracts and excluded 1,487. Of 94 full text articles reviewed, we included 9. Four articles were added from our hand search of reference lists resulting in a total of 27 references included for human resource practices (Key Question #1).

We identified 541 abstracts pertaining to organizational culture. After excluding 497, we reviewed 44 full text articles and included 2. One article was added from the specific team-based care search and 6 articles were added from hand searching resulting in a total of 9 included references.

The physical environment search resulted in 49 abstracts. We excluded 46 and reviewed the full text of 3 articles. All 3 were excluded. The 2 articles included in the report were added after hand searching.

Figure 3. Literature Flow Diagram – Human Resource Practices Studies

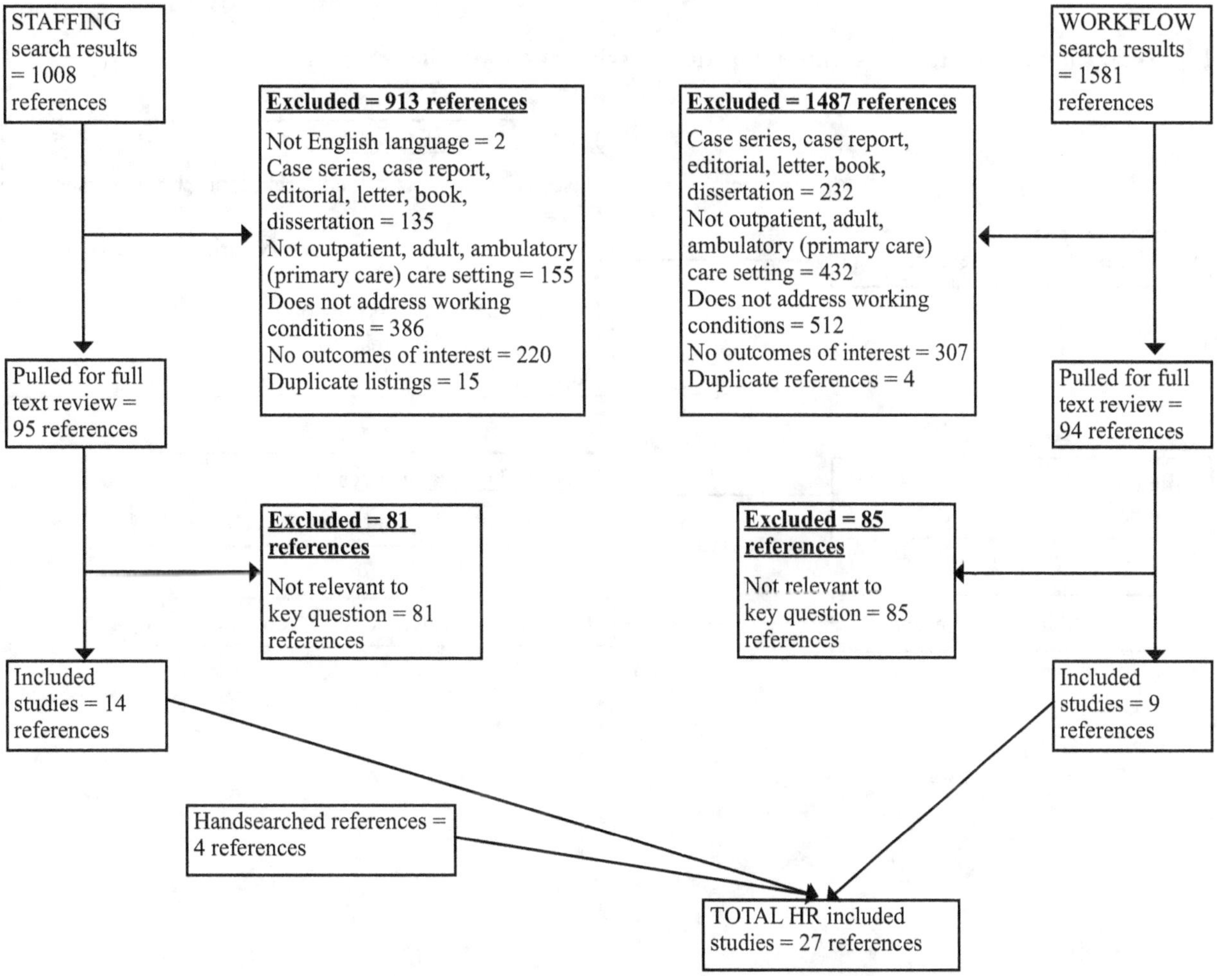

Figure 4. Literature Flow Diagram – Organizational Culture Studies

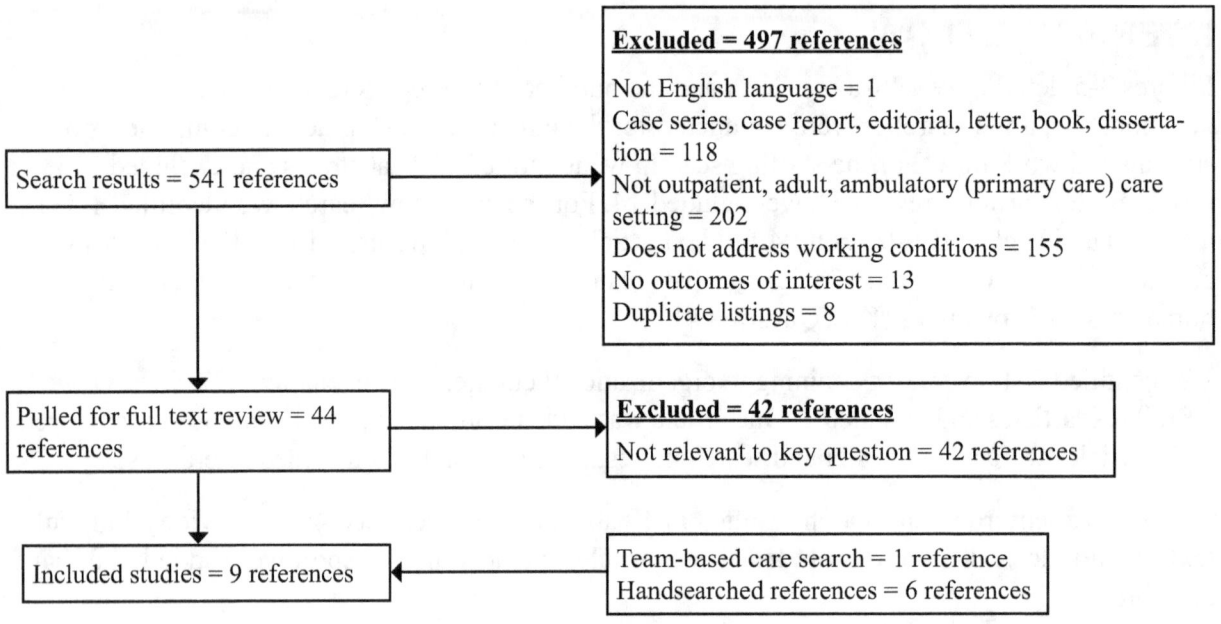

Figure 5. Literature Flow Diagram – Physical Environment Studies

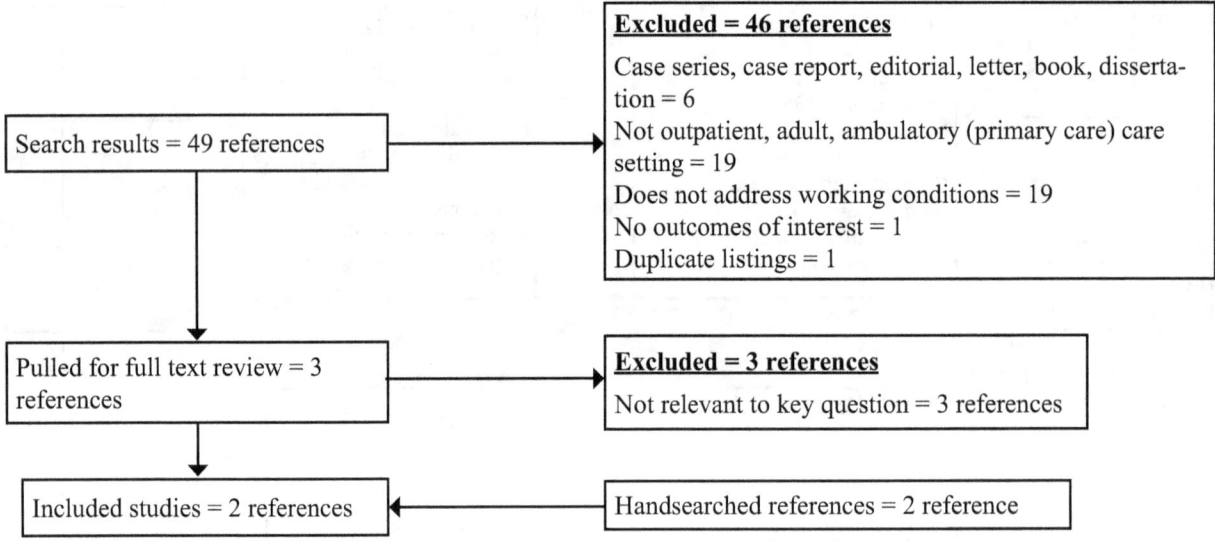

KEY QUESTION #1. How are human resource practices, such as skill levels, training, workload, hours worked, autonomy, and electronic medical records/systems, associated with patient outcomes?

   a. quality of care (access and effectiveness)
   b. safety (medication errors)
   c. patient satisfaction (with provider, with clinic/practice)

Twenty-seven studies (12 set in the US, 13 set in Europe, and 2 set outside of the US/Europe) met inclusion criteria.[6, 32-57] We summarize these studies in Appendix D, Tables 1-3. In Table 1, we present an overall summary of studies by HR practice and patient outcome studied. We reviewed studies that investigated the following HR practices a) skills (measured as MD versus NP or PA skill level), b) training (different training interventions to increase patient communication, visit efficiency or clinical effectiveness), c) workload (measured most often as the provider's listsize), d) hours (measured as either full time versus part time work, as a continuous measure of hours worked, or hours worked after being on-call), e) autonomy (provider report of control over work tasks), and f) electronic medical records (EMR) system or other computerized system (e.g., referral system). We discuss the main findings for each HR practice below.

The Effect of Working Conditions on Patient Care: A Systematic Review

Table 1. Human Resource Practices Studies by HR Practice Studied and Patient Outcome Studied

HR Practice Studied	First Author, Year	Quality of Care: Clinical Effectiveness or Access	Patient Safety: Reduced Errors[1]	Patient Satisfaction: With Provider	Patient Satisfaction: With Practice or Care
Skills	Caldow 2006[32]	n/a	n/a		↔
Skills	Dierick-van Daele 2009[33]	n/a	n/a	↔	
Skills	Laurant 2008[34]	n/a	n/a	→	
Skills	Mundinger 2000*[35]	n/a	n/a	↔	
Skills	Roblin 2004*[36]	n/a	n/a	→	↔
Training	Castro 2009*[37]			↔	
Training	Edwards 2004[38]			↔	
Training	Goulet 2007[39]	↑			
Training	Haas 2006*[40]			↔	
Training	Zabar 2010*[41]	↑		↔	
Workload	Campbell 2001[42]	→			
Workload	Campbell 2005[43]	→			
Workload	Carlsen 2006[44]			↔	
Workload	Dong 2010[45]		↑		
Workload	Grytten 2009[46]				↔
Workload	Linzer 2009*[6]	↔	↔		
Workload	Luras 2007[47]			↑	←
Workload	Magan 2011[48]	→			
Workload[2]	Nyweide 2009*[49]	↑			
Workload	Salisbury 2010[50]			↔	↔
Hours	Fairchild 2001*[51]	→		↔	↔
Hours	French 2001[52]			↔	↔
Hours	Parkerton 2003*[53]	→		↔	
Autonomy	Linzer 2009*[6]	↔	←	↔	
Autonomy	McKinstry 2007[54]				→
EMR	DesRoches 2008*[55]	←	←		→
EMR	Feldstein 2010*[56]	←			
EMR[3]	Weiner 2009*[57]	←			
Total Studies[4]		12	3	14	7

*Indicates the study was conducted in the U.S. [1]This outcome has been reverse coded in this table so that a positive effect (up arrow) indicates the study found a *reduction* in medical errors. [2]Measured as Medicare caseload in this study. [3]EMR refers to an electronic referral system in this study. [4]This is a count of the total number of unique studies that evaluate each patient outcome. There are 27 total studies that evaluate at least one HR practice and one patient outcome. An "up" arrow indicates that the presence/implementation of an HR practice (training, autonomy, EMR) or the increase in a practice (skill level, workload, or hours) was associated with higher quality of care, more reduced errors (i.e., better patient safety), or greater patient satisfaction. A "down" arrow indicates that increasing/implementing the HR practice resulted in lower quality of care, fewer reduced errors, or less patient satisfaction. The ↔ arrow indicates that no significant association was found.

Skills

Two US and three European studies were included that focused on how provider skill level (MD vs. NP/PA) influenced patient satisfaction. Overall, the evidence was inconsistent on the effect of provider skill level on patient satisfaction. One large cross-sectional study of over 26,000 Kaiser Permanente patients in Georgia found that patients were about 15 percent ($p<0.05$) more likely to be satisfied with the provider interaction received when seeing a PA/NP instead of an MD, but found no significant difference in satisfaction with care by skill level of the provider,[36] as did one smaller scale cross-sectional study set in the Netherlands.[34] However, two studies where patients were randomly assigned to either an MD or an NP found no evidence of differences in patient satisfaction by skill level.[33,35] We identified one VA study that examined patient satisfaction scores from 1.6 million veterans seen in 21 VISNs and reported aggregate changes in patient satisfaction over time by VISN, but the authors did not report these results stratified by skill level except for three specific VISNs where satisfaction increased when more NP/PAs were hired,[58] so we were unable to include this study in our review. Overall, the evidence was inconsistent on the effect that provider skill level has on patient satisfaction. We do note that the two randomized control studies found no effect. Following the 2003 AHRQ report, we did not review studies that examined the effect of skill levels on patient quality of care or patient safety as it is widely accepted that medical school or more training increases quality of care.[4]

Training

Five studies (three US, one Canadian, and one European) were included that evaluated the effectiveness of a training intervention on patient satisfaction and quality of care. All four that examined patient satisfaction found no effect of various training programs. These training programs included training on how to effectively structure visits,[40] communication skills workshops,[41] shared decision making and risk communication training,[38] and a provider report of having received cultural competence training.[37] The latter study was not an analysis of the intervention and only examined correlations between provider report of having received cultural competence training and patient satisfaction (i.e., no pre/post analysis).[37] However, two studies (one US and one Canadian study) found a positive effect of training (communication skills workshop and a remedial professional development program) on clinical effectiveness measured from audits of patient charts for guideline concordant care.[39,41] Overall, we find some evidence that training might improve clinical effectiveness, but little evidence that it affects patient satisfaction. There were no studies included in our review that examined the effect of training on patient safety, in this case medication errors; however, there is a large literature investigating the role of training on patient safety in hospital settings (e.g., surgical training) that has found, in general, that more training improves patient safety (e.g., Wachter, 2004;[2] Shapiro et al., 2004[59]).

Workload

Ten studies were included that investigated how provider workload affects patient outcomes. Three of the four studies (all European) that specifically examined patient satisfaction found no correlation between workload and patient satisfaction. However, the measures of patient satisfaction in two of these studies included satisfaction with wait time or ability to get an appointment.[46,50] Only one study found a positive correlation between provider workload and patient satisfaction measured specifically as satisfaction with the care received.[47] Thus, we conclude that there is little evidence that workload affects patient satisfaction with the provider, though it might influence satisfaction with the ability to get an appointment.

Three of the five studies (one US and three European) found that workload negatively affects quality of care, measured as guideline concordant care for management of chronic conditions,[42] access to provider,[43] and rates of ambulatory care sensitive hospitalizations.[48] One study reported that care quality scores were not significantly different for providers with high time pressure or for those who worked in a "chaotic office."[6] The fifth study reported that greater Medicare caseloads were needed to obtain higher rates of patients getting preventive care screening.[49] However, as that study uses a different measure of workload (which may arguably not be a good proxy for workload), we conclude that there is some evidence suggesting that higher workloads negatively influence quality of care.

Finally, two studies (one in the US and one in China) investigated workload and patient safety. The US study surveyed almost 1,800 patients across 119 clinics in 5 urban and rural area and found that a greater workload (time needed per patient divided by the time allotted per patient) had no effect on non-medication treatment errors assessed from chart audits.[6] However, a large study of over 20,000 prescriptions written from 680 primary care clinics in rural China found that physicians with greater workloads (patient visits/month) were about 70 percent more likely to prescribe 5 or more drugs per patient than those with lighter workloads.[45] Thus, given that these studies are not representative and yield conflicting findings, we conclude that there is insufficient evidence about the role of workload on patient safety. However, as discussed in the previous paragraph, two studies found no effect of workload on guideline concordant care and one found no effect on ambulatory care sensitive hospitalizations, all of which could be considered measures of patient safety.

Hours

Three studies (two US and one European) were included that investigated how provider work hours affects patient satisfaction and quality of care. All three studies found no effect of providers' work hours on patient satisfaction; regardless of whether hours were measured as full time vs. part-time (less than 30 hours per week),[51] as a continuous measure of appointment hours,[53] or designated as hours surrounding "on call" versus "off call" duty.[52] However, two of these studies also examined the effect of hours on patient quality of care and found that providers who work fewer hours were more likely to be compliant with guidelines for preventive care screening and management of a chronic disease.[51,53] Thus, based on these three studies, our review suggests that while provider's work hours may not have influenced patient satisfaction, there was some preliminary evidence that longer work hours may have negatively affected quality of care provided. We note that most of these studies meet few of the low risk of bias quality criteria described in the Appendix. There were no studies included in our review that investigated hours and patient safety (in this case, medication errors), though there is a large literature examining the effect of hours worked among nurses, residents and in hospital settings (see AHRQ report[4]).

Autonomy

Two studies (one US and one European) were included that investigated provider reports of autonomy, or provider control over work tasks, and patient outcomes. The Linzer et al., study (described above),[6] found that providers who reported greater control (based on a 14 item scale that was then dichotomized) did not have greater quality "scores" based on chart audits assessing their management of chronic conditions but did have lower error "scores" based on chart audits assessing their missed treatment opportunities, inattention to behavioral factors and guideline non-adherence. A study based in Scotland found that patients were less satisfied with how they were treated by staff and wait time for visits where the provider reported greater control of work.[54] Although these two studies are suggestive, this is insufficient evidence to draw conclusions about the role of job autonomy on patient outcomes.

Electronic Medical Records

Three studies (all US) were included that investigated EMRs or other computerized systems that affected how providers do their jobs. All three studies found that EMR systems improved quality of care by alerting providers to critical lab values, assisting providers to provide preventive care, order lab work, tests, or specialty referrals.[55-57] One study also found evidence that an EMR system that gave warnings and clinical decision support was more effective in helping providers prevent drug allergies or dangerous medication interactions over more basic systems without those capabilities.[55] While these three studies suggest that EMR systems have improved patient quality of care, one study relied on provider reports of how the system aided work, as opposed to more objective measures.[55] One large study utilized panel data methods to assess specialty referrals before and after an electronic medical referral system was put in place,[57] but the other two studies relied on cross-sectional or cohort analysis. Thus, the evidence is suggestive that EMR systems improve patient quality, but more intervention analyses should be done and there is insufficient evidence on how EMR systems affect patient satisfaction.

Pay for Performance

One theoretical component of workplace conditions is the practice of Pay for Performance (P4P) where providers are partially compensated with incentive payments based on quality of care. A large body of literature focused on P4P exists, but we discuss two more recent systematic reviews without doing a systematic review of the P4P literature.[60,61] Although Christianson et al.[60] reported improvement in select quality measures, they also concluded that the role of financial incentives for providers in quality improvement is unclear. The authors underlined variation in targeted outcomes, criteria for incentives, and questions based on provider reactions to incentives as topics for further research. A 2010 review of one hundred twenty-eight evaluation studies[61] made similar conclusions. Thus, while there may be some evidence of the effectiveness of P4P systems, two recent systematic reviews conclude that there is too much variation in the evidence, study designs, and provider attributes to make clear conclusions about the effect of P4P on patient outcomes.

Summary of Findings

We identified three randomized controlled trials, seven longitudinal (cohort or pre-post with repeated cross-sections) studies, and 17 cross-sectional studies investigating the role of HR practices in primary care clinics in explaining patient outcomes.

Nine of eleven studies we examined that focused on patient quality of care as an outcome, specifically measured clinical effectiveness, thus there is insufficient evidence on the role of provider workplace conditions on access as a quality of care measure. The most frequently studied HR practice for quality of care was workload and, in general, the evidence suggests that an increased workload results in lower quality of care. However, the only two US studies found either no effect[6] or a positive effect.[49] Furthermore, all of the workload studies were cross-sectional and often were not low risk of bias studies. The other HR practices studied were evaluated less frequently, but there was more consistency in the results across studies: more training (2 studies), shorter hours (2 studies), and computerized systems (3 studies) lead to better quality. Only one study we reviewed examined provider autonomy or flexibility and found mixed effects on quality of care scores; this is insufficient evidence for the role of autonomy. Overall, these results are suggestive but make it difficult to make strong conclusions about the role of HR practices on patient quality of care.

We identified three studies in our review that explicitly examined the role of workplace conditions on patient safety, measured as medication errors, in the primary care setting. While these were relatively well designed studies, more studies are needed. Because only two studies examined workload, one examined autonomy and one examined computerized systems, there is insufficient evidence to answer our key question about how HR practices influence patient safety.

We identified 17 unique studies that investigated how HR practices influence patient satisfaction with either the provider or the clinic. We found mixed evidence on the role of provider skills (MD vs. NP/PA) on patient satisfaction; two studies found no effect and two cross-sectional studies found a negative effect of skills. We also found mixed evidence on the role of provider workload with one study finding a positive effect and two finding no effect. All four of the studies that examined provider training and all three that examined provider work hours found that they had no effect on patient satisfaction. Overall, there is suggestive evidence that training and work hours do not effect patient satisfaction, but again, because of the lack of studies, we cannot make strong conclusions about these findings. Similarly, we conclude that there is inconsistent evidence on the role of skills and workload. We identified no studies that looked at how computerized systems affect patient satisfaction.

Quality of Evidence for Key Question #1

Quality of randomized and non-randomized trials was assessed as described in the Methods section. Items considered in assessing the quality of randomized trials are presented with the study description (Appendix D, Tables 1-3). Figure 6 depicts the percent of the non-randomized trials that met the criteria for each quality dimension assessed.

Figure 6. Study Quality of Human Resource Practices Non-Randomized Studies

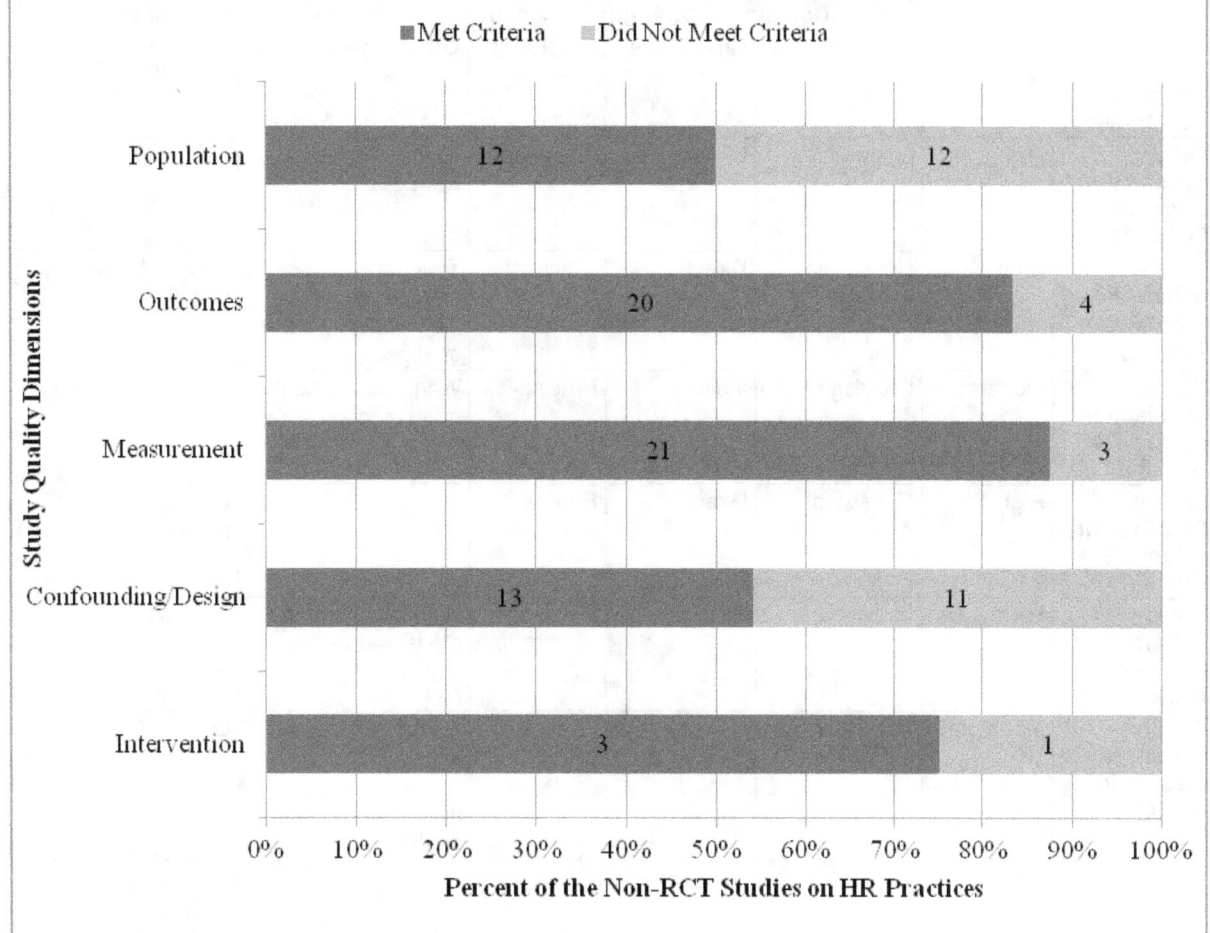

Notes: There were 24 (out of 27) non-RCT studies examining HR practices and patient outcomes. Only 4 of these studies included intervention (and thus were evaluated on that dimension). The numbers on each bar indicate the number of studies that either met the study quality criteria (dark gray) or did not (light gray).

We evaluated the strength of evidence for the workplace conditions and patient outcomes for which we had at least three studies (Table 2). Strength of evidence overall was low for patient satisfaction and provider skills, workload, and hours; and for quality of care and provider workload and electronic medical records. Most of the evidence was rated high or moderate on risk of bias due to the lack of many well-designed RCTs or observational studies that address potential biases. There was also inconsistent measurement of both the workplace condition constructs and the patient outcome constructs, which made comparisons across studies difficult. There was insufficient evidence for patient safety and all workplace conditions, quality of care and training and hours, and patient satisfaction and EMR. Additionally, there was insufficient evidence on provider autonomy and all patient outcomes.

Table 2. Human Resource Practices – Strength of Evidence for Key Outcomes

Workplace Condition & Patient Outcome (# of studies)	Domains of Strength of Evidence					Overall Strength of Evidence (SOE) (effect if consistent)
	Risk of Bias	Consistency	Directness	Precision	Other Notes	
Patient Satisfaction & Provider Skills (5)	High	Inconsistent	Direct	Imprecise		Low SOE
Patient Satisfaction & Provider Training (4)	High	Consistent	Direct	Precise	Training is measured inconsistently across studies	Low SOE (positive effect)
Patient Satisfaction & Provider Workload (4)	Moderate	Consistent	Indirect	Precise	Workload is often measured as "listsize"	Low SOE (no effect)
Patient Satisfaction & Provider Hours (3)	High	Consistent	Direct	Precise		Low SOE (no effect)
Quality of Care & Provider Workload (5)	High	Inconsistent	Indirect	Precise	Workload is often measured as "listsize"	Low SOE
Quality of Care & Electronic Medical Records (3)	Moderate	Consistent	Indirect	Precise	EMR/computerized systems are measured inconsistently across studies	Low SOE (positive effect)

KEY QUESTION #2. How are other working conditions, such as organizational culture or physical environment, associated with patient outcomes?

> a. quality of care (access and effectiveness)
> b. safety (medication errors)
> c. patient satisfaction (with provider, with clinic/practice)

Organizational Culture

Nine studies met inclusion criteria.[6,62-69] Six studies were conducted in the United States and three in Canada. We summarize study characteristics in Appendix D, Table 7. We reviewed studies that examined the following four organizational culture components: a) patient-centered medical homes (PCMH) (patient-centered approach to care management and coordination through a practice based care team), b) team-based care (multi-disciplinary care centered around the primary care physician to facilitate communication among care team members), c) care environment (environment and culture focused on delivering care to a specific demographic of the population), and d) clinic values (perceptions of how organizational values line up with personal values of providers). Table 3 provides an overview of the distribution of studies by reported outcomes (quality of care, patient safety, patient satisfaction, and provider outcomes).

PCMH

Two pre-post observational studies reported quality of care outcomes based on the organizational culture component of PCMH.[63,64] Both studies showed improvements in quality of care at clinics where PCMH was implemented. Although Reid et al. found no improvement in hospitalization rates for PCMH clinics compared with usual care, PCMHs resulted in significant improvements in hospitalizations for ambulatory care sensitive conditions (ACSC).[64] The second study demonstrated significant improvement in hospital admission and readmission rates for PCMH clinics against modeled controls.[63] Reid et al.[64] also found that patient satisfaction with provider (quality of interaction, shared decision making, coordination of care, access to provider) and care (patient involvement, goal setting/tailoring) increased after the implementation of PCMH. Although there were only two studies reviewed, both employed a pre-post observational design and suggested that PCMH improved quality of care and patient satisfaction.

Team-based Care

Five studies reported outcomes for the primary care cultural component of team-based care.[65-69] Three studies evaluated the effect of team based care on quality of care outcomes.[65,67,68] Two of these studies, including one randomized controlled trial,[68] found that team based care significantly increased quality of care, measured as chronic disease management and preventive care with the use of team care[68] and patient rated quality of life.[67] However, the third study, a case-control design, demonstrated no change in hospitalizations or emergency room (ER) visits.[65] Two studies evaluated patient satisfaction with team-based care[65,66] and found mixed results. One cross-sectional study showed no improvement in patient satisfaction,[65] whereas the randomized controlled trial study found a two-fold increase in patient rating of chronic care for team-based guided care versus usual care.[66] Finally, one study randomized 48 physicians and their patients to receive pharmacists' consultations or usual care and found that face-to-face patient-pharmacist consultations identified at least one drug problem in 79 percent of the intervention population with no data provided for control physicians.[69] Overall, these studies present contradictory evidence making it difficult to make conclusions about how effective team-based primary care is for improving quality of care or patient satisfaction. We identified only one study that evaluated the effect of teams on patient safety in the ambulatory care setting,[69] but comparison data were not presented in this study.

Care Environment

We reviewed one cross sectional study that reported patient satisfaction with care based on the care environment.[62] Specifically, among women using the Veterans Health Administration (VHA) system of care, attending a women's clinic was a significant positive predictor for all measures of patient satisfaction with care (privacy and comfort, communication, complete care, follow-up, receiving care, overall) when compared with usual primary care clinics. This one study is insufficient to make conclusions about the role of the care environment on patient satisfaction. We identified no studies that investigated the relationship between the care environment and quality of care or patient safety.

Clinic Values

One cross-sectional study looked at clinic values in relation to provider satisfaction, and quality of care.[6] The study found a positive association between clinical values such as quality emphasis, information and communication emphasis, organizational trust, workplace cohesiveness, and values alignment and total quality measured by diabetes care, hypertension management, and preventive care. Thus, there is insufficient evidence on the role of clinic values or norms in explaining patient outcomes.

Table 3. Organizational Culture Studies by Practice Studied and Patient Outcome Studied

Practice Studied	First Author, Year	Quality of Care — Clinical Effectiveness or Access	Patient Safety — Reduced Errors	Patient Satisfaction — With Provider	Patient Satisfaction — With Practice or Care
Care environment	Bean-Mayberry 2003*[62]				↑
Clinic Values	Linzer 2009*[6]	↑			
PCMH	Gilfillan 2010*[63]	↑			
PCMH	Reid 2009*[64]	↑		↑	↑
Team-based care	Adam 2010*[65]	↔			↔
Team-based care	Boyd 2009*[66]				↑
Team-based care	Chomienne 2011[67]	↑			
Team-based care	Hogg 2009[68]	↑			
Team-based care	Sellors 2003[69]		↔		
Total studies[1]		6	1	1	4

*Indicates the study was conducted in the U.S.

[1]This is a count of the total number of unique studies for each outcome. There are 8 total studies that evaluate at least one organizational culture practice and one patient outcome. An "up" arrow indicates that the increase in /implementation of an organizational culture practice was associated with higher quality of care, more reduced errors (i.e., better patient safety), or greater patient satisfaction. A "down" arrow indicates that increasing/implementing the organizational practice resulted in lower quality of care, fewer reduced errors, or less patient satisfaction. The ↔ arrow indicates that no significant association was found.

Summary of Findings for Organizational Culture

There is limited evidence from two pre-post quasi-experimental studies on PCMH as a primary care cultural component. These studies reported positive effects of PCMHs on quality of care, and the one study that evaluated the effect of PCMH on patient satisfaction found a positive effect. We conclude that there is suggestive evidence that PCMHs increase quality of care, but in general insufficient evidence on the effect of PCMHs on patient outcomes. PCMH studies were assessed to have a high risk of bias meeting only two of five quality criteria for non-randomized studies as described in the methods section.

Limited data from five studies provided inconsistent evidence that team-based care improved quality, patient safety, or patient satisfaction. Two studies found positive effects of team-based care and patient quality of care, however one of these was a high risk of bias study. The other study on quality of care and teams found no effect. Thus, while the evidence is suggestive that team-based care improves patient quality of care, more well-designed studies are needed. Results for patient satisfaction were unclear as one cluster-randomized controlled trial with a low risk of bias reported that patients seen by guided care teams had twice greater odds of rating chronic care highly[66] and one cross-sectional study found no significant association. Finally, results for patient safety or medication errors are inconclusive for team-based care due to limited evidence from one randomized controlled trial with a high risk of bias[69] that did not report comparison effects.

Evidence for the effect of care environment on patient satisfaction is also unclear. One cross sectional study which met one of four quality criteria for non-randomized controlled trials showed higher patient satisfaction with care among women attending a women's clinic at the Veterans Health Administration. Related studies investigating the effect of "clinic values" and quality of care suggested a positive correlation with quality of care. However, validated measures of the care environment or clinic values are needed in order to make comparisons across studies.

Strength of Evidence for Organizational Culture

The strength of evidence for the affect of PCMH on quality of care is low primarily due to a high risk of bias, and inconsistencies in reported effect size. The studies directly related PCMH interventions to quality of care without surrogates, but a rating of precision was not applicable due to lack of pooled outcomes. Only one study reported on patient satisfaction with PCMH therefore the body of evidence is insufficient for strength assessment.

The strength of evidence for the effect of team-based care on quality of care is low due to studies with a high risk of bias, inconsistencies in the reported effect sizes, and indirect reporting using surrogate measures for quality of care. Again, a rating of precision was not applicable due to lack of pooled outcomes. Only one study reported on patient safety with team-based care and therefore the body of evidence is insufficient. The strength of evidence for the effect of team-based care on patient satisfaction is low due to studies with a high risk of bias, an indirect link to patient satisfaction, and inconsistent effect sizes. A measure of precision was not applicable. The evidence for the effect of care environment or clinic values on quality of care or patient satisfaction is insufficient as each component of organizational culture included only one study.

Figure 7. Study Quality of Organizational Culture Non-Randomized Studies

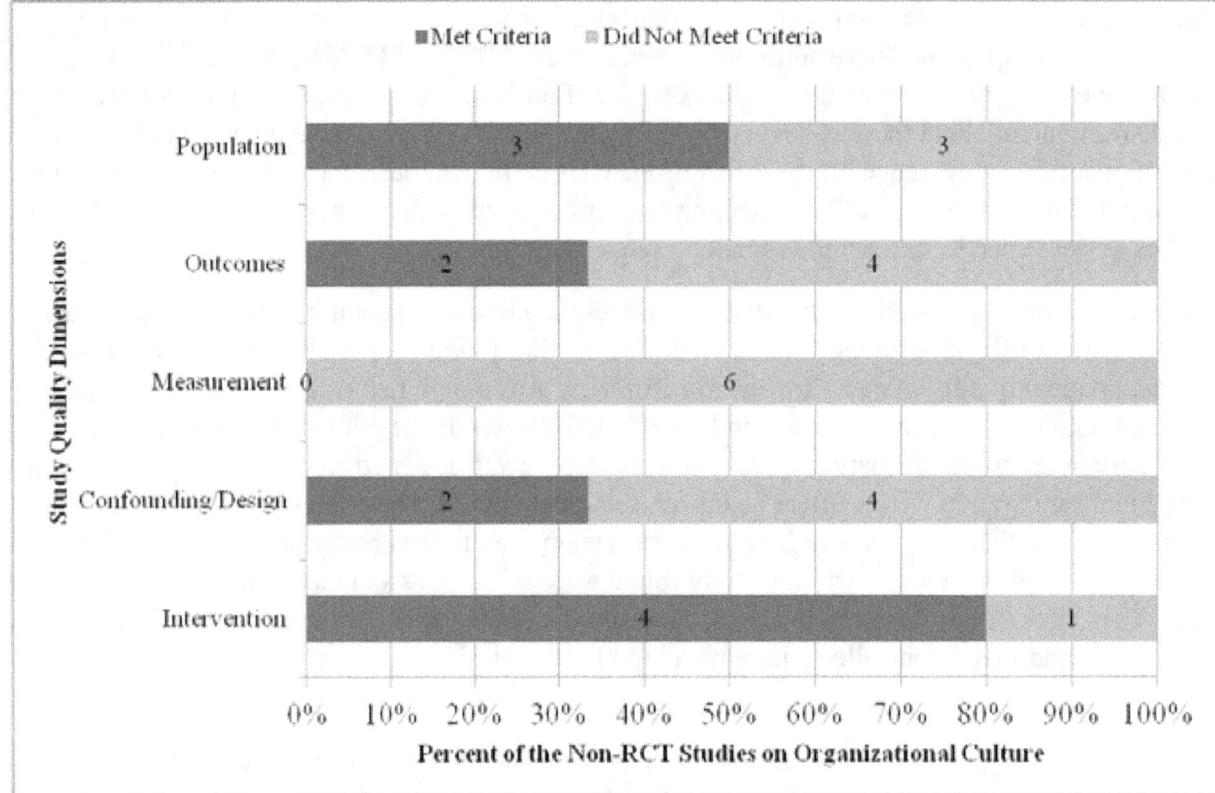

Notes: There were 6 (out of 9) non-RCT studies examining organizational culture practices and patient outcomes. Only 5 of 6 studies provided outcomes based on interventions. The numbers on each bar indicate the number of studies that either met the study quality criteria (dark gray) or did not (light gray).

Physical Environment

Two studies met inclusion criteria[70,71] are summarized in Appendix D, Table 12. One study was conducted in the United States[71] and one was conducted in the United Kingdom (UK).[70] We also present data from a systematic review of patient satisfaction with electronic health record (EHR) use in examination rooms.

Table 4. Physical Environment Studies by Patient Outcome Studied

	Quality of Care	Patient Safety	Patient Satisfaction	
First Author, Year	Clinical Effectiveness or Access	Reduced Errors	With Provider	With Practice or Care
Arneill 2002[71]	↑*			↑**
Rice 2008[70]				↑

*Study measured "perceived" quality of care; **Study measured "perceived" comfort in environment
An "up" arrow indicates that "better" physical environment was associated with higher quality of care or greater patient satisfaction

The UK study evaluated patient anxiety and satisfaction and patient-doctor communications before and after relocating to a new clinic facility.[70] Enhanced environmental features of the new clinic included lighting, sound, space, privacy, furnishings, and artwork. Patients reported significantly less anxiety both before and after a provider consultation in the new facility (Table 5). They also preferred the new reception/waiting area and consultation rooms and rated satisfaction with doctor-patient communication higher in the new facility.

Table 5. Physical Environment Outcomes[70]

Variable	Phase 1 (pre-move)	Phase 2 (post-move)	Significance
STAI Pre-consultation[a]	11.7	10.9	$p<0.001$
STAI Post-consultation[a]	10.5	10.1	$p=0.03$
Reception/Waiting Area Rating[b]	33.3	39.8	$p<0.001$
Consultation Room Rating[c]	23.0	26.7	$p<0.001$
Communication with Provider Rating[d]	37.6	38.5	$p=0.003$

[a]STAI=Spielberger State-Trait Anxiety Inventory, range of scores 6 to 24; [b]range 9-45; [c]range 6-30; [d]range 6-42; [e]range 0-12

In the US study, participants were asked to view and rate slide images of clinic waiting rooms.[71] The slides were from 28 waiting rooms and included clinics in renovated houses, in office buildings, and connected to hospitals. The rooms varied in size, color, lighting, and furnishings. A factor analysis found that perceived quality of care was higher for waiting rooms rated high on "attractive lighting" and "colorful and neat" and lower for waiting rooms rated as "unusual-looking." There were differences between the college student and the senior citizen groups and a significant gender by number of office visits interaction. The factor analysis for comfort in the environment found that people were more comfortable in waiting rooms described as "tasteful" or "decorative" and less comfortable in waiting rooms described as "dark and sparse" or "strange and uncomfortable." There were differences between the college students and senior citizens and between men and women. Although clinic waiting rooms are not, by strict definition, provider working areas, we have included this study as it presents patient perceptions of the overall clinic environment.

A systematic review of seven studies assessing patient satisfaction with the use of EHRs in the exam room during visits with providers found mixed results.[72] The authors noted methodological problems with the studies. Pooled results from 3 studies indicated higher patient satisfaction following the introduction of EHRs in the exam rooms (mean difference of 3.7%). One of the studies included in the review was done in a VA primary care clinic. That study found that patients seeing residents were more likely to report a negative effect of the EHR on the patient-physician interaction but that only 8% of patients thought that the computer interfered with their relationship with their physician.

Summary of Findings for Physical Environment
The available evidence suggests that physical environment can affect patients' anxiety levels before and after their appointments, satisfaction with doctor-patient communications, and

perceived quality of care. However, additional research is needed to determine the specific elements of the environment that influence these outcomes and whether environment may also have an effect on additional outcomes such as patient safety and quality of care.

Quality and Strength of Evidence for Physical Environment

The percentage of studies meeting quality criteria for non-randomized trials is shown in Figure 8. With only one study reporting actual patient satisfaction there is insufficient evidence for this outcome.

Figure 8. Study Quality of Physical Environment Non-Randomized Studies

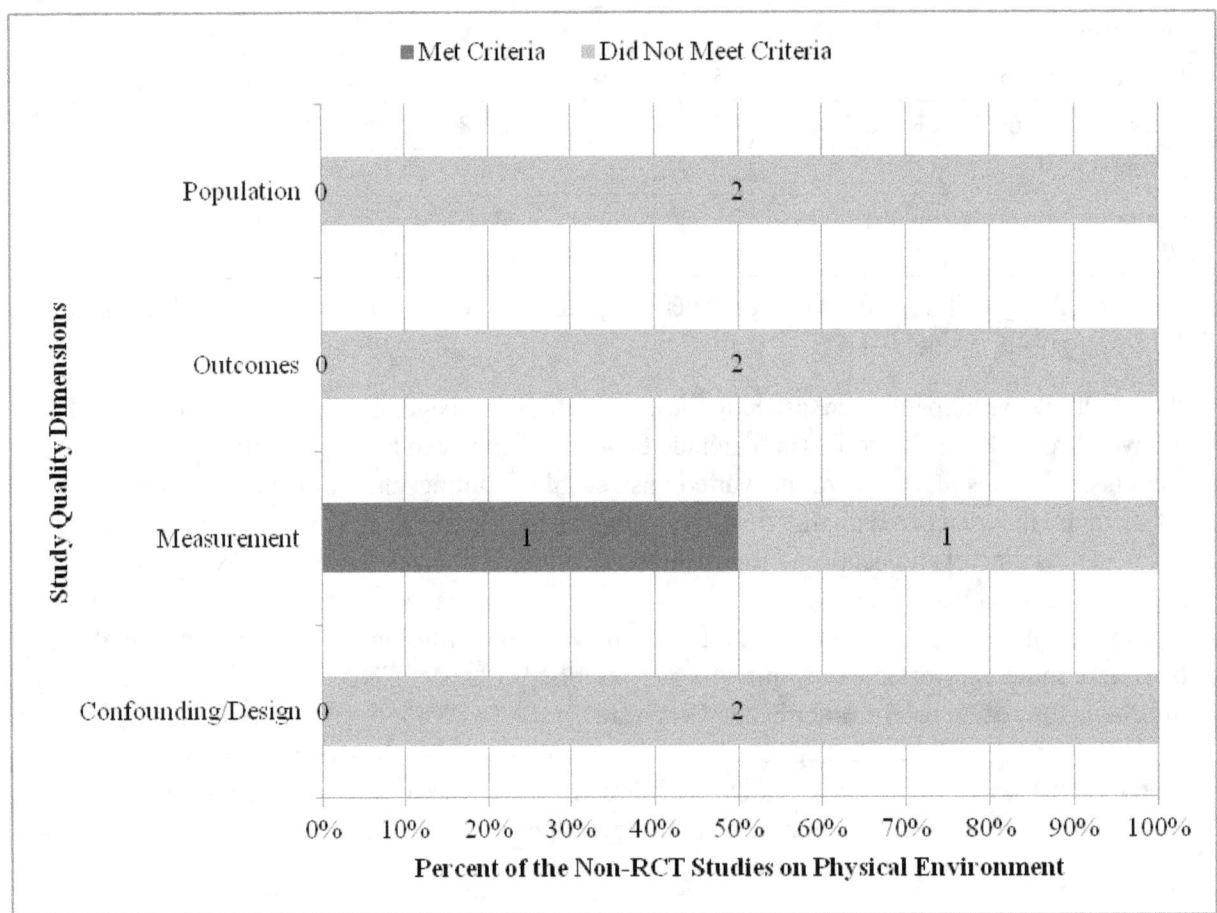

Notes: Only one study involved an intervention and the study did not meet the quality criteria for an intervention. The numbers on each bar indicate the number of studies that either met the study quality criteria (dark gray) or did not (light gray).

KEY QUESTION #3. In studies that report provider outcomes, how are working conditions associated with provider outcomes (e.g., job satisfaction, productivity, pay)?

As noted in the background and conceptual model sections, we do not systematically review the evidence on the intermediate link between workplace conditions and provider outcomes. However, among the studies included in our review for evidence on the role of workplace condition on patient outcomes, three (two US and one European) also report findings on provider outcomes. We discuss those findings here, noting that these results are not necessarily representative of the evidence published to date on provider outcomes and workplace conditions in primary care settings. Linzer and colleagues[6] found that greater workloads and less job autonomy resulted in greater physician ratings of stress and burnout and lower ratings of job satisfaction. They also found evidence that certain aspect of organizational culture (e.g. trust, quality emphasis, workplace cohesion) had similar affects on provider outcomes. The other US study of approximately 2,700 MDs from the 2007 American Medical Association file found that job satisfaction was not affected by the use of more advanced electronic medical records systems as compared to more basic systems.[55] One study found that providers had higher levels of stress when working after a night "on call" compared to working after a night of not being on duty.[52]

In addition to the study by Linzer et al.[6] reported above, two other organizational culture studies reported provider outcomes.[64,67] In one study, physicians and physician assistants at PCMH clinics reported significantly lower emotional exhaustion.[64] In the second study, physicians reported that office atmosphere, quality of life at work, and workload all improved when psychologists were integrated into family practice.[67]

One study of physical environment also reported limited provider outcome data.[70] Staff members expressed significantly greater work satisfaction in a new facility but there were no differences in psychological symptoms. They felt the new work environment was more professional and allowed them to provide improved service to patients

SUMMARY AND DISCUSSION

SUMMARY OF EVIDENCE BY KEY QUESTION

Key Question #1

We identified three randomized controlled trials, seven longitudinal (cohort or pre-post with repeated cross-sections) studies and 17 cross-sectional studies investigating the role of HR practices in primary care clinics in explaining patient outcomes.

Nine out of eleven of the studies we examined that focused on patient quality of care as an outcome, specifically measured clinical effectiveness, thus there is insufficient evidence on the role of provider workplace conditions on access as a quality of care measure. The most frequently studied HR practice for quality of care was workload and while three of the studies suggested that an increase in workload results in lower quality of care, one study also found a positive effect and one found no effect. The other HR practices studied were evaluated less frequently, but there was more consistency in the results across studies: more training (2 studies), shorter hours (2 studies), and computerized systems (3 studies) lead to better quality. Only one study we reviewed examined provider autonomy or flexibility and found mixed effects on quality of care scores; this is insufficient evidence for the role of autonomy. Overall, these results are suggestive but make it difficult to make strong conclusions about the role of HR practices on patient quality of care.

We identified three studies in our review that explicitly examined the role of human resource practices on patient safety in the primary care setting. While these were relatively well designed studies, more studies are needed. Because only two studies examined workload, one of which also examined autonomy, and the third study examined computerized systems, there is insufficient evidence to answer our key question about how HR practices influence patient safety.

We identified 17 unique studies that investigated how HR practices influence patient satisfaction with either the provider or the clinic. We found mixed evidence on the role of provider skills (MD vs. NP/PA) on patient satisfaction; two studies found no effect and two studies found a negative effect of skills. We found mostly no effect of provider workload on patient satisfaction (3 studies), with the exception of one Norwegian study reporting that a longer listsize resulted in greater patient satisfaction. All four of the studies that examined provider training and all three that examined provider work hours found that they had no effect on patient satisfaction. Thus, there was suggestive evidence that training and work hours do not effect patient satisfaction, but again because of the lack of well-designed studies, we cannot make strong conclusions about these findings. Similarly, we conclude that there is inconsistent evidence on the role of skills and workload. We identified no studies that looked at how electronic medical records or computerized systems affect patient satisfaction.

Key Question #2

The available literature provides low strength or insufficient evidence for varied components of organizational culture including PCMH, team-based care, care environment, and clinic values and their effect on outcomes highlighted in our key questions. Such evidence does not permit conclusions with regard to quality of care, patient safety, and patient satisfaction.

Our report on the influence of organizational culture parallels a systematic review published by the Cochrane Collaboration in 2011 titled "The Effectiveness of Strategies to Change Organizational Culture to Improve Healthcare Performance."[73] The report considered any strategy intended to change organizational culture in order to improve healthcare performance. While the Cochrane review identified similar outcomes of interest (quality of care, patient satisfaction, organizational performance, and provider outcomes), no studies met their inclusion criteria. The Cochrane review was not limited to ambulatory primary care settings, but sought only studies meeting quality criteria developed by the Cochrane Effective Practice and Organisation of Care Group (EPOC). While our review used a similar definition of organizational culture, we included a broader range of methodologies.

The 2003 AHRQ review[4] looked at the effect of organizational culture on measures of patient safety. The authors discussed difficulty in examining the affect of cultural factors on patient outcomes rooted in the broadly defined concepts ranging from cultural norms, to more concrete practice interventions. Their report concluded that despite multiple studies using diverse study methodologies conducted in different workplace settings, there was insufficient evidence related to the effect of organizational factors on patient safety. Similarly, our report found insufficient evidence across diverse constructs of organizational culture to draw conclusions related to quality of care, patient safety, and patient satisfaction.

Although there has been research on the effect of physical environment (notably lighting, color, auditory stimuli, and temperature) on workplace performance, much of that work has been done in industrial settings and what has been done in healthcare has largely focused on hospitals.[4,74] We found few studies that examined the effect of physical environment in primary care clinics. No study attempted to isolate any one component of the physical environment. Reported outcomes focused on patient self-report of anxiety and satisfaction with no objective measures of patient safety, quality of care, or provider performance.

Key Question #3

Consistent with more thorough systematic reviews of the literature examining how workplace conditions affect providers' stress, job satisfaction, etc., among the studies in our review that also examined provider outcomes, we found that greater workloads and less control over work tasks resulted in greater provider stress, burnout, and job satisfaction. One study we examined found that electronic medical records did not result in greater provider stress.

The relationships between workplace conditions, provider outcomes, and patient outcomes are complex and dynamic in such a way that not only are the effects felt at many levels (provider, patient, healthcare system), but also they create a cycle of reinforcing behaviors and outcomes. There are several potential policy interventions at the various levels that might positively influence provider wellbeing. In this study, we focus on studies that shed light on possible workplace interventions (as opposed to provider self-care or higher-order system level interventions) that will ultimately impact patient outcomes. Such changes to workplace conditions will likely also influence provider outcomes. However, we present these results as only suggestive, but consistent with other literature, including systematic reviews, that has established evidence on the intermediate link between workplace conditions and provider outcomes.

RECOMMENDATIONS FOR FUTURE RESEARCH

As shown in Tables 1, 3, and 4, there is little research that investigates the effects of working conditions on patient safety, which we measure specifically as medication errors, in the primary care setting. More generally, more well-designed studies are needed to replicate the few that have been conducted. For example, all ten of the studies we reviewed that investigated the role of workload were cross-sectional studies. While undertaking randomized controlled trials may be impractical, well-designed cohort studies or other pre-post designs will allow for more convincing evidence on the causal effect of the workplace conditions.

Additionally, there is a need for research that looks rigorously at the interdependent role of human resource practices (such as hours worked, provider autonomy, and electronic medical records), organizational culture, and physical environment in explaining patient outcomes in primary care settings. Research on the role of workplace conditions in explaining worker productivity, turnover, burnout, and other employee outcomes suggests that many of these characteristics are "bundled"[75-77] and complementary. For example, a clinic that rolls out team-based care will likely also have other workplace conditions and workflow designs that facilitate teamwork, such as electronic medical records or an organizational culture that values teamwork. However, none of the studies we reviewed investigated how the "system" or complete workplace environment affected patient outcomes. Studying the effect of one HR practice, such as electronic medical records or teams, ignores the fact that these practices occur within a larger organizational setting with a particular organizational culture and related or complementary practices. Thus, isolating the marginal effect of just one of these practices is empirically difficult. Larger scale studies that are able to compare more clinics or hospitals and more fully characterize the workplace are needed.

The development of or more consistent use of construct valid measures of both working conditions and patient or provider outcomes in the primary care settings is needed to make comparisons across studies easier. Future research should incorporate randomized controlled trials or high quality quasi-experimental designs.

CONCLUSIONS

Overall, the studies we reviewed suggest that in primary care settings:

- a lighter provider workload/shorter work hours, more provider training, and computerized systems result in higher patient quality of care
- provider training and work hours have no effect on patient satisfaction.

We find mixed evidence on the effect of provider skill levels and workload on patient satisfaction. We identified very few studies in our review that explicitly examined the role of workplace conditions on patient safety or the role of the physical environment on patient outcomes in the primary care setting, thus more studies are needed. Several workplace conditions have been insufficiently studied and thus there is no evidence on how these practices matter in ambulatory care settings: the effect of computerized systems, provider autonomy and teams on patient satisfaction; and the effect of autonomy on quality of care. We also note that the lack of evidence does not necessarily imply the lack of a relationship; we also do not explore other possible hypotheses, including the possibility that workplace conditions affect healthcare providers, but healthcare providers are still able to do their jobs adequately such that patients are not affected.

The available literature provides low strength or insufficient evidence for varied components of organizational culture including PCMH, team-based care, care environment, and clinic values and their effect on outcomes highlighted in our key questions. Such evidence does not permit conclusions with regard to quality of care, patient safety, and patient satisfaction.

We found two studies that focused on the effect of physical environment in primary care clinics. No study attempted to isolate any one component of the physical environment. Reported outcomes included self-report of anxiety and satisfaction with no objective measures of patient safety or quality of care.

Consistent with more thorough systematic reviews of the literature examining how workplace conditions affect providers' stress, job satisfaction, etc., among the studies in our review that also examined provider outcomes, we found that greater workloads and less control over work tasks resulted in greater provider stress, burnout, and less job satisfaction. One study we examined found that electronic medical records did not result in greater provider stress.

REFERENCES

1. Institute of Medicine. *To Err is Human: Building a Safer Health System.* Washington, D.C.: National Academy Press, 2000.

2. Wachter RM. The end of the beginning: patient safety five years after 'To Err Is Human'. *Health Affairs.* 2004;23:534-545.

3. Wachter RM. Patient safety at ten: unmistakable progress, troubling gaps. *Health Affairs.* 2010;29(1),165-173.

4. Hickam DH, Severance S, Feldstein A, et al. The effect of health care working conditions on patient safety. Evidence Report/Technology Assessment Number 74. (Prepared by Oregon Health & Science University under Contract No. 290-97-0018.) Rockville, MD: Agency for Healthcare Research and Quality, 2003.

5. Baron RJ, Fabens EL, Schiffman M, Wolf E. Electronic health records: just around the corner? or over the cliff? *Ann Intern Med.* 2005;143:222-6.

6. Linzer M, Manwell LB, Williams ES, et al. Working conditions in primary care: physician reactions and care quality. *Ann Intern Med.* 2009;151(1):28-36.

7. Hauer KE, Durning SJ, Kernan WN, et al. Factors associated with medical students' career choices regarding internal medicine. *JAMA* 2008;300(10):1154-64.

8. Bodenheimer T, Grumbach K, Berenson RA. A lifeline for primary care. *N Engl J Med.* 2009;360:2693-6.

9. Wallace JE, Lemaire JB, Ghali WA. Physician wellness: a missing quality indicator. *Lancet* 2009;374:1714-21.

10. Stone PW, Harrison MI, Feldman P, et al. Organizational climate of staff working conditions and safety-an integrative model. In Henriksen K, Battles JB, Marks ES, Lewin DI (eds.) *Advances in Patient Safety: From Research to Implementation (Vol. 2: Concepts and Methodology).* Rockville, MD: Agency for Healthcare Research and Quality, 2005.

11. Warren N, Hodgson M, Craig T, Dyrenforth S, Perlin J, Murphy F. Employee working conditions and healthcare system performance: the Veterans Health Administration experience. *J Occup Environ Med.* 2007;49:417-429.

12. Donabedian A. Evaluating the quality of medical care. *Milbank Mem Fund Q.* 1966;44:166-206.

13. Mitchell PH, Lang NM. Framing the problem of measuring and improving healthcare quality: has the quality health outcomes model been useful? *Med Care.* 2004;42:II4-11.

14. Campbell SM, Roland MO, Buetow SA. Defining quality of care. *Soc Sci Med.* 2000;51:1611-25.

15.   Elder N, Dovey SM. Classification of medical errors and preventable adverse events in primary care: A synthesis of the literature. *J Fam Pract*. 2003;51:927-32.

16.   Sitzia J, Wood N. Patient satisfaction: a review of issues and concepts. *Soc Sci Med*. 1997;45(12):1829-43.

17.   Parker PA, Kulik JA. Burnout, self- and supervisor-rated job performance, and absenteeism among nurses. *J Behav Med*. 1995;18(6):581-599.

18.   Shader K, Broome ME, Broome CD, West ME, Nash M. Factors influencing satisfaction and anticipated turnover for nurses in an academic medical center. *J Nurs Admin*. 2001;31(4):210-216.

19.   Williams ES, Skinner AC. Outcomes of physician job satisfaction: A narrative review, implications, and directions for future research. *Health Care Manage Rev*. 2003;28(2):119-40.

20.   Williams ES, Manwell LB, Konrad TR, Linzer M. The relationship of organizational culture, stress, satisfaction, and burnout with physician-reported error and suboptimal patient care: results from the MEMO study. *Health Care Manage Rev*. 2007;32(3):203-12.

21.   Devoe J, Fryer GE, Hargraves JL, Phillips RL, Green LA. Does career dissatisfaction affect the ability of family physicians to deliver high-quality patient care? *J Fam Pract*. 2002;51(3):223-8.

22.   Haas LJ, Glazer K, Houchins J, Terry S. Improving the effectiveness of the medical visit: a brief visit-structuring workshop changes patients' perceptions of primary care visits. *Patient Educ Couns*. 2006;62(3):374-8.

23.   McKevitt C, Morgan M, Dundas R, Holland WW. Sickness absence and 'working through' illness: a comparison of two professional groups. *J Public Health Med*. 1997;19:295–300.

24.   Jones JW, Barge BN, Steffy BD, Fay LM, Kunz LK, Wuebker LJ. Stress and medical malpractice: organizational risk assessment and intervention. *J Appl Psychol*. 1988;73:727-35.

25.   Shanafelt TD, Bradley KA, Wipf JW, Back AL. Burnout and self reported patient care in an internal medicine residency program. *Ann Intern Med*. 2002;136:358–67.

26.   Fahrenkopf AM, Sectish TC, Barger LK, et al. Rates of medication errors among depressed and burnt out residents: prospective cohort study. *BMJ*. 2008;336:488–91.

27.   Misra-Hebert AD, Kay R, Stoller JK. A review of physician turnover: rates, causes, and consequences. *Am J Med Qual*. 2004;19:56-66.

28.   West CP, Huschka MM, Novotny PJ, et al. Association of perceived medical errors with resident distress and empathy: a prospective longitudinal study. *JAMA* 2006;296:1071–78.

29.   Sirriyeh R, Lawton R, Gardner P, Armitage G. Coping with medical error: a systematic review of papers to assess the effects of involvement in medical errors on healthcare professionals' psychological well-being. *Qual Saf Health Care.* 2010;19:e43.

30.   Higgins JPT, Green S (eds). *Cochrane Handbook for Systematic Reviews of Interventions.* Version 5.0.2 [updated September 2009]. The Cochrane Collaboration, 2009. Available at www.cochrane-handbook.org. Accessed August 29, 2011.

31.   Owens DK, Lohr KN, Atkins D, et al. AHRQ series paper 5: grading the strength of a body of evidence when comparing medical interventions--agency for healthcare research and quality and the effective health-care program. *J Clin Epidemiol.* 2010;63:513-23.

32.   Caldow J, Bond C, Ryan M, et al. Treatment of minor illness in primary care: a national survey of patient satisfaction, attitudes and preferences regarding a wider nursing role. *Health Expect.* 2007;10(1):30-45.

33.   Dierick-van Daele AT, Metsemakers JF, Derckx EW, Spreeuwenberg C, VrijhoefHJ. Nurse practitioners substituting for general practitioners: randomized controlled trial. *J Adv Nurs.* 2009;65(2):391-401.

34.   Laurant MG, Hermens RP, Braspenning JC, Akkermans RP, Sibbald B, Grol RP. An overview of patients' preference for, and satisfaction with, care provided by general practitioners and nurse practitioners. *J Clin Nurs.* 2008;17(20):2690-8.

35.   Mundinger MO, Kane RL, Lenz ER, et al. Primary care outcomes in patients treated by nurse practitioners or physicians: a randomized trial. *JAMA.* 2000;283(1):59-68.

36.   Roblin DW, Becker ER, Adams EK, Howard DH, Roberts MH. Patient satisfaction with primary care: does type of practitioner matter? *Med Care.* 2004;42(6):579-90.

37.   Castro A, Ruiz E. The effects of nurse practitioner cultural competence on Latina patient satisfaction. *J Am Acad Nurse Pract.* 2009;21(5):278-86.

38.   Edwards A, Elwyn G, Hood K, et al. Patient-based outcome results from a cluster randomized trial of shared decision making skill development and use of risk communication aids in general practice. *Fam Pract.* 2004;21(4):347-54.

39.   Goulet F, Gagnon R, Gingras M-E. Influence of remedial professional development programs for poorly performing physicians. *J Contin Educ Health Prof* 2007;27(1):42-8.

40.   Haas JS, Cook EF, Puopolo AL, Burstin HR, Cleary PD, Brennan TA. Is the professional satisfaction of general internists associated with patient satisfaction? *J Gen Intern Med.* 2000;15(2):122-8.

41.   Zabar S, Hanley K, Stevens DL, et al. Can interactive skills-based seminars with standardized patients enhance clinicians' prevention skills? Measuring the impact of a CME program. *Patient Educ Couns.* 2010;80(2):248-52.

42.   Campbell JL, Ramsay J, Green J. Practice size: impact on consultation length, workload, and patient assessment of care. *Br J Gen Pract.* 2001;51 (469):644-50.

43.   Campbell JL, Ramsay J, Green J, Harvey K. Forty-eight hour access to primary care: practice factors predicting patients' perceptions. *Fam Pract.* 2005;22(3):266-8.

44.   Carlsen B, Aakvik A. Patient involvement in clinical decision making: the effect of GP attitude on patient satisfaction. *Health Expect.* 2006;9(2):148-57.

45.   Dong L, Van H, Wang D. Polypharmacy and its correlates in village health clinics across 10 provinces of Westem China. *J Epidemiol Community Health.* 2010;64(6):549-53.

46.   Grytten J, Carlsen F, Skau I. Services production and patient satisfaction in primary care. *Health Policy.* 2009;89(3):312-21.

47.   Luras H. The association between patient shortage and patient satisfaction with general practitioners. *Scand J Prim Health Care.* 2007;25(3):133-9.

48.   Magan P, Alberquilla A, Otero A, Ribera 1M. Hospitalizations for ambulatory care sensitive conditions and quality of primary care: their relation with socioeconomic and health care variables in the Madrid regional health service (Spain). *Med Care.* 2011;49(1): 17-23.

49.   Nyweide DJ, Weeks WB, Gottlieb DJ, Casalino LP, Fisher ES. Relationship of primary care physicians' patient caseload with measurement of quality and cost performance. *JAMA.* 2009;302(22):2444-50.

50.   Salisbury C, Wallace M, Montgomery AA. Patients' experience and satisfaction in primary care: secondary analysis using multilevel modelling. *BMJ.* 2010;341:c5004.

51.   Fairchild DG, McLoughlin KS, Gharib S, et al. Productivity, quality, and patient satisfaction: comparison of part-time and full-time primary care physicians. *J Gen Intern Med* 2001;16(10):663-7.

52.   French DP, McKinley RK, Hastings A. GP stress and patient dissatisfaction with nights on call: an exploratory study. GP stress and patient satisfaction. *Scand J Prim Health Care.* 2001;19(3):170-3.

53.   Parkerton PH, Wagner EH, Smith DG, Straley HL. Effect of part-time practice on patient outcomes. *J Gen Intern Med* 2003;18(9):717-24.

54.   McKinstry B, Walker J, Porter M, et al. The impact of general practitioner morale on patient satisfaction with care: a cross-sectional study. *BMC Fam Pract.* 2007;8:57.

55.   DesRoches CM, Campbell EG, Rao SR, et al. Electronic health records in ambulatory care--a national survey of physicians. *N Engl J Med.* 2008;359(1):50-60.

56.   Feldstein AC, Perrin NA, Unitan R, et al. Effect of a patient panel-support tool on care delivery. *Am J Manag Care.* 2010;16(10):e256-66.

57.   Weiner M, El Hoyek G, Wang L, et al. A web-based generalist-specialist system to improve scheduling of outpatient specialty consultations in an academic center. *J Gen Intern Med.* 2009;24(6):710-5.

58.   Budzi D, Lurie S, Singh K, Hooker R. Veterans' perceptions of care by nurse practitioners, physician assistants, and physicians: a comparison from satisfaction surveys. *J Am
Acad Nurse Pract.* 2010;22(3):170-6.

59.   Shapiro MJ, Morrey J, Small SD, et al. Simulation based teamwork training for emergency department staff: does it improve clinical team performance when added to an existing
didactic teamwork curriculum? *Qual Saf Health Care.* 2004;13(6):417-21.

60.   Christianson JB, Leatherman S, Sutherland K. Lessons from evaluations of purchaser
pay-for-performance programs. *Med Care Res Rev.* 2008;65(6 Suppl):5S-35S.

61.   Van Herck P, De Smedt D, Annemans L, Remmen R, Rosenthal M, Sermeus W. Systematic review: Effects, design choices, and context of pay-for-performance in health care.
BMC Health Serv Res. 2010;10(1):247.

62.   Bean-Mayberry BA, Chang CC, McNeil MA, Whittle J, Hayes PM, Scholle SH. Patient
satisfaction in women's clinics versus traditional primary care clinics in the Veterans Administration. *J Gen Intern Med* 2003;18(3):175-81.

63.   Gilfillan RJ, Tomcavage J, Rosenthal MB, et al. Value and the medical home: effects of
transformed primary care. *Am J Manag Care.* 2010;16(8):607-14.

64.   Reid RJ, Fishman PA, Yu O, et al. Patient-centered medical home demonstration:
a prospective, quasi-experimental, before and after evaluation. *Am J Manag Care.*
2009;15(9):e71-87.

65.   Adam P, Brandenburg DL, Bremer KL, Nordstrom DL. Effects of team care of frequent
attenders on patients and physicians. *Fam Syst Health.* 2010;28(3):247-57.

66.   Boyd CM, Reider L, Frey K, et al. The effects of guided care on the perceived quality of
health care for multi-morbid older persons: 18-month outcomes from a cluster randomized controlled trial. *J Gen Intern Med.* 2010;25(3):235-42.

67.   Chomienne M-H, Grenier J, Gaboury I, Hogg W, Ritchie P, Farmanova-Haynes E. Family
doctors and psychologists working together: doctors' and patients' perspectives. *J Eval
Clin Pract.* 2011;17(2):282-7.

68.   Hogg W, Lemelin J, Dahrouge S, et al. Randomized controlled trial of anticipatory and
preventive multidisciplinary team care: for complex patients in a community-based primary care setting. *Can Fam Physician.* 2009;55(12):e76-85.

69.   Sellors J, Kaczorowski J, Sellors C, et al. A randomized controlled trial of a phar-
macist consultation program for family physicians and their elderly patients. *CMAJ.*
2003;169(1):17-22.

70.   Rice G, Ingram J, Mizan J. Enhancing a primary care environment: a case study of effects
on patients and staff in a single general practice. *Br J Gen Pract.* 2008;58(552):465-70.

71.   Arneill AB, Devlin AS. Perceived quality of care: the influence of the waiting room environment. *J Environ Psychol.* 2002;22(4):345-60.

72. Irani JS, Middleton JL, Marfatia R, Omana ET, D'Amico F. The use of electronic health records in the exam room and patient satisfaction: a systematic review. *J Am Board Fam Med.* 2009;22:553-62.

73. Parmelli E, Flodgren G, Schaafsma ME, Baillie N, Beyer FR, Eccles MP. The effectiveness of strategies to change organizational culture to improve healthcare performance. *Cochrane Database Syst Rev* 2011, Issue 1. Art. No.: CD008315.

74. Gulwadi GB, Joseph A, Keller AB. Exploring the impact of the physical environment on patient outcomes in ambulatory care settings. *HERD.* 2009;2(2):21-41.

75. Ichniowki C, Shaw K, Prennushi G. The effects of human resource management practices on productivity: working paper. New York: Columbia University, 1994.

76. Huselid MA. The impact of human resource management practices on turnover, productivity, and corporate financial performance. *Acad Manage J.* 1995;38(3):635-72.

77. MacDuffie JP. Human resource bundles and manufacturing performance: flexible production systems in the world auto industry. *Indus Lab Rel Rev.* 1995;48:197-221.

APPENDIX A. SEARCH STRATEGIES

Staffing

Database: Ovid MEDLINE(R)

----

1   exp Medical Errors/
2   (medical errors or medication errors or diagnostic errors).mp.
3   quality of health care/
4   *safety/ or safety/st or safety management.mp.
5   Iatrogenic Disease/ or iatrogenic disease.mp.
6   quality assurance health care/
7   (patient safety or safety of patient$).mp.
8   *treatment outcome/
9   Patient$.ti
10 exp Physician-Patient Relations/
11 exp Patient Satisfaction/
12 or/1-11
13 workload/ or workload.mp. or overwork.mp.
14 exp professional competence/
15 work schedule tolerance/ or teamwork.tw.
16 "Personnel Staffing and Scheduling"/ or personnel staffing.mp.
17 Professional Autonomy/ or professional autonomy.mp.
18 professional power.mp.
19 exp Time Management/
20 or/13-19
21 12and 20
22 limit 21to (english language and humans) 23 limit 22 to yr="2000 -Current"
24 exp Physicians/
25 exp Nurse Practitioners/
26 exp Physician Assistants/
27 or/24-26
28 23 and 27
29 limit 28 to (comment or editorial or letter or news)
30 28 not 29

Workflow

Database: Ovid MEDLINE(R)

----

1   exp Medical Errors/
2   (medical errors or medication errors or diagnostic errors).mp.
3   quality of health care/
4   *safety/ or safety/st or safety management.mp.
5   Iatrogenic Disease/ or iatrogenic disease.mp.
6   quality assurance health care/
7   (patient safety or safety of patient$).mp.
8   *treatment outcome/
9   Patient$.ti.
10 exp Physician-Patient Relations/
11 exp Patient Satisfaction/

12 or/1-11
13 exp Efficiency, Organizational/
14 exp "Task Performance and Analysis"/
15 exp Information Systems/
16 exp Electronic Health Records/
17 exp Equipment Design/
18 exp Equipment Safety/
19 Personnel Management/ or job performance.mp.
20 exp User-Computer Interface/
21 exp Expert Systems/
22 (distraction or interruption).mp.
23 multitask.mp.
24 paging.mp.
25 User-Computer Interface/ or human computer interactions.mp.
26 exp "Referral and Consultation"/
27 or/13-26
28 12 and 27
29 limit 28 to (english language and humans)
30 limit 29 to yr="2000-Current"
31 exp physicians/
32 exp nurse practitioners/ \33   exp physician assistants/
34 or/31-33
35 30 and 34
36 limit 35 to (comment or editorial or letter or news)
37 35 not 36

Organizational culture

Database: Ovid MEDLINE(R)

----

1   exp Medical Errors/
2   (medical errors or medication errors or diagnostic errors).mp.
3   quality of health care/
4   *safety/ or safety/st or safety management.mp.
5   Iatrogenic Disease/ or iatrogenic disease.mp.
6   quality assurance health care/
7   (patient safety or safety of patient$).mp.
8   *treatment outcome/
9   Patient$.ti.
10 exp Physician-Patient Relations/
11 exp Patient Satisfaction/
12 or/1-11
13 exp Interprofessional Relations/ or exp Organizational Culture/ or professional culture.mp.
14 organizational climate.mp.
15 exp Leadership/
16 management style.mp.
17 managerial style.mp.
18 skill mix.mp.

19 exp Models, Organizational/ or shared leadership.
    mp. or exp Organizational Innovation/
20 open door policies.mp.
21 exp Management Quality Circles/
22 exp Institutional Management Teams/
23 or/13-22
24 12 and 23
25 limit 24 to (english language and humans)
26 limit 25 to yr="2000 -Current"
27 exp physicians/
28 exp nurse practitioners/
29 exp physician assistants/
30 or/27-29
31 26 and 30
32 limit 31 to (comment or editorial or letter or news)
33 31 not 32

Physical environment

Database: Ovid MEDLINE(R)
----

1   exp Medical Errors/
2   (medical errors or medication errors or diagnostic
    errors).mp
3   quality of health care/
4   *safety/ or safety/st or safety management.mp.
5   Iatrogenic Disease/ or iatrogenic disease.mp.
6   quality assurance health care/
7   (patient safety or safety of patient$).mp.
8   *treatment outcome/
9   Patient$.ti.
10 exp Physician-Patient Relations/
11 exp Patient Satisfaction/
12 or/1-11
13 exp Air Pollution/
14 exp Air Pollution, Indoor/
15 exp Light/ or exp Lighting/ or indoor lighting.mp.
16 exp Acoustics/
17 exp Noise/ or indoor noise.mp.
18 exp "Interior Design and Furnishings"/
19 exp Humidity/
20 exp Ventilation/ or exp Temperature/ or indoor
    temperature.mp. or exp Environmental Monitoring/
21 exp "Facility Design and Construction"/ or clinic
    design.mp
22 human factors engineering.mp.
23 exp Environment Design/ or facility environment.
    mp.
24 or/13-23
25 12 and 24
26 limit 25 to (english language and humans)
27 limit 26 to yr="2000-Current"
28 exp physicians/
29 exp nurse practitioners/
30 exp physician assistants/

31 or/28-30
32 27 and 31
33 limit 32 to (comment or editorial or letter or news)
34 32 not 33

Team

Database: Ovid MEDLINE(R)
----

1   exp Patient Care Team/ or team-based.mp.
2   practice based care team.mp.
3   shared case.mp.
4   exp Interprofessional Relations/ or shared care.mp.
5   collaborative care.mp.
6   multidisciplinary care teams.mp.
7   multidisciplinary care team.mp.
8   6 or 7
9   or/1-8
10 exp Medical Errors/
11 (medical errors or medication errors or diagnostic
    errors).mp.
12 quality of health care/
13 *safety/ or safety/st or safety management.mp.
14 Iatrogenic Disease/ or iatrogenic disease.mp.
15 quality assurance health care/
16 (patient safety or safety of patient$).mp.
17 *treatment outcome/
18 Patient$.ti.
19 exp Physician-Patient Relations/
20 exp Patient Satisfaction/
21 or/10-20
22 9 and 21
23 limit 22 to (english language and humans)
24 limit 23 to yr="2000 -Current"
25 exp Physicians/
26 exp Nurse Practitioners/
27 exp Physician Assistants/
28 or/25-27
29 24 and 28
30 limit 29 to (comment or editorial or letter or news)
31 29 not 30

APPENDIX B. CRITERIA USED IN QUALITY ASSESSMENT OF NON-RANDOMIZED STUDIES

We evaluated each non-randomized trial based on the five elements below. To be considered low risk of bias for any element, a "yes" response was required for each of the questions (a, b, c) pertaining to the element, if applicable. Plots were developed to show the percent of the non-randomized trials in each area (human resources practices, organizational culture, and physical environment) that were assigned a yes (met criteria) or no (failed to meet criteria) for each element.

1) **Population**

   a. Is the sample representative of the population of interest?
   b. Did researchers apply inclusion/exclusion criteria uniformly to all comparison groups and is the selection of the comparison group appropriate?
   c. Is the sampling method appropriate (i.e. appropriate database or sample for research question, adequate response rate for survey studies, etc.)?

2) **Outcomes**

   a. Are important outcomes assessed and *reported* (i.e. not just intermediate or surrogate outcomes)?
   b. Was the length of follow-up appropriate for the research questions (consider benefits and harms)?
   c. Is the impact of loss to follow-up (or differential loss to follow-up) considered in the analysis?

3) **Measurement**

   a. Are outcome, predictor and covariates assessed in the same way for everyone?
   b. Is this blinded such that, for example, a person's exposure status would not be known at the time outcome status was assessed? This is where recall bias and other types of differential assessment come into play.
   c. Are the tools used to assess exposures and outcomes accurate and reliable (i.e., are standard measures used)?

4) **Confounding**

   a. Are the statistical methods and study design adequate for minimizing confounding?
   b. Aside from the exposure of interest, are groups balanced in terms of factors that might bias the exposure and outcome association?
   c. Are the appropriate confounding factors included in the analysis?

5) **Intervention (if applicable)**

   a. Is the intervention clearly described and transferrable (i.e. could someone else repeat this study with different staff and patients and get similar results)?

APPENDIX C. PEER REVIEW COMMENTS/AUTHOR RESPONSES

REVIEWER COMMENT	RESPONSE
1. Are the objectives, scope, and methods for this review clearly described?	
Yes	No response needed
Yes, articulate and concise	No response needed
Yes	No response needed
Yes	No response needed
Yes. Well designed and conceptualized with appropriate questions to guide the review. Excellent use of criteria for literature search and review of the literature.	Thank you.
The rationale for choosing these 3 areas specifically: HR, organizational culture, and physical environment probably warrants some enhancement. Further, the definitions and limits of each of these categories seems somewhat arbitrary. For example, would sufficient staffing to ensure a appropriate roles/functions for team based care be considered HR or organizational culture? Regarding outcomes, you use the term patient safety, but it is often unclear that you really mean to include all quality metrics including typical clinical outcomes such as admissions and ED utilization. What about performance metrics such as chronic disease outcomes such as glycemic control etc?? I am still not sure if you included these as well.	We acknowledge that these categorizations are arbitrary, but we do not think that how we've organized this (by the categorizations that we've used) undermines our presentation of the evidence, which in most cases is lacking. Our main rationale for using these categorizations is that we wanted to build on the previous similar AHRQ report, but because of the substantial overlap collapsed a few of the categories. Nonetheless, we've inserted a disclaimer about this categorization.

Regarding patient safety, this is a valid point. We agree that there may be some overlap with patient safety and effectiveness (which we point out in the report), where the latter would include "performance metrics such as chronic disease outcomes such as glycemic control etc." We have added some discussion to clarify this. |
2. Is there any indication of bias in our synthesis of the evidence?	
No	No response needed
No	No response needed
No	No response needed
No	No response needed
No Good description of algorithm for choosing studies. Excellent use of criteria for quality of review and for systematic reporting of findings.	Thank you.
No	No response needed
3. Are there any <u>published</u> or <u>unpublished</u> studies that we may have overlooked?	
No	No response needed
It appears that a thorough literature review was conducted; however I have not done my own lit search on this topic to know if there are additional references	No response needed

45

The Effect of Working Conditions on Patient Care: A Systematic Review

REVIEWER COMMENT	RESPONSE
Here are a few suggestions: 1. Williams ES, Konrad TR, Linzer M, et al. Physician, Practice, and Patient Characteristics Related to Primary Care Physician Physical and Mental Health: Results from the Physician Worklife Survey. Health Serv Res 2002;37(1):121-143. 2. Clarke SP, Rockett JL, Sloane DM, et al. Organizational climate, staffing, and safety equipment as predictors of needlestick injuries and near-misses in hospital nurses. Am J Infection Control 2002;30(4):207-216 3. Aiken L, Clarke S, Sloane D, et al. Hospital nurse staffing and patient mortality, nurse burnout, and job dissatisfaction. JAMA 2002;288:1987–1993. 4. Needleman J, Buerhaus P, Mattke S, et al. Nurse-staffing levels and the quality of care in hospitals. NE Journal of Medicine 2002;346(22):1715–1722. 5. Stone PW, Harrison ML, Feldman P, et al. Organizational Climate of Staff Working Conditions and Safety—An Integrative Model. Advances in Patient Safety: From Re-search to Implementation. Volumes 1-4, AHRQ Publication Nos. 050021 (1-4). February 2005. Agency for Healthcare Research and Quality, Rockville, MD. http://www.ahrq.gov/qual/advances/ Volume 2, Concepts & Methodology, pp 467-481 These basic references/syntheses do not appear in the citations, but the first is mentioned on page 10, just not referenced. 1. Institute of Medicine. To Err is Human: Building a Safer Health System. Washington, DC: National Academy of Sciences; 2000. 2. Institute of Medicine. Crossing the Quality Chasm: A New Health System for the 21st Century. Washington, DC: National Academy of Sciences; 2001. 3. Institute of Medicine Committee on the Work Environment for Nurses and Patient Safety. Keeping Patients Safe: Transforming the Work Environment of Nurses. Ann Page, Editor. Washington DC: National Academy of Sciences; 2004.	Thank you for the additional suggested articles. We've pulled all of these references and discuss them here: 1. Williams et al. – this article does not have any patient outcomes that we examine so it does not meet our inclusion criteria. However, the study does relate well to some of our discussion of provider outcomes, so we will make sure this paper is added/discussed in that section. 2. Clarke et al. – this article does not meet our inclusion criteria because it is about needlesticks in hospital settings and deals with nurses' workplace condition (while we focus on MDs, PAs, and NPs only). 3. Aiken et al - this article does not meet our inclusion criteria because it deals with hospital settings and nurses' workplace condition (while we focus on MDs, PAs, and NPs only in primary care settings). 4. Needleman et al – same as #3. 5. Stone et al – we will add this citation to our background/framework section. We only cite the first Institute of Medicine report. We have changed the citation from Kohn et al. to Institute of Medicine.
No If there are other studies, I am not aware of them in the prescribed area of interest. There are studies looking at the effects of working conditions and workload of nurses.	No response needed
No Literature with data/results that I am familiar with has made it into this report.	No response needed

4. Additional suggestions or comments	
While the report concludes that the evidence of an association of working conditions with health care outcomes is often lacking, alternative hypotheses are not explicitly entertained. It may be that health professionals are capable of "buffering" pateints from the effects of adverse working conditions, leading to null or mixed effects.	We have added this caveat.
None, excellent work	Thank you.

Comment	Response
p. 5 – 5th paragraph under Conclusions. The first sentence seems to indicate greater job satisfaction is associated with greater workloads and less control over work tasks. The sentence reads " …we found that greater workloads and less control over work tasks resulted in greater provider stress, burnout, and job satisfaction." I would suggest some rewording if this is not the intent.	Re pg. 5, 5th paragraph: we've edited this. Re pg. 38: we've added some discussion.
Page 38 – Recommendations for Future Research. This section was weak in comparison to the rest of the report. The content is very general with little specific direction or suggestion of priority areas for future research. Given the focus on general healthcare reform and the budget constraints what we are facing in the VA, the authors may want to speculate on some specific areas or research questions that need addressing to help us prepare for tough times ahead. Are there specific practices or aspects of culture or of the physical environment that their findings would point to as logical next steps for research?	
Thank you for the opportunity to review this report. I appreciated the detail and the clarity of presentation. This type of work is important as we advance this area of knowledge.	
It seems that there would be much overlap between HR, org culture, and physical environment. It is hard to know if some studies may have been overlooked because of the vagueness of these terms. This review will be helpful more to point out the limitations of the current literature, and the lack of clear relationship observed thus far between team staffing, training and function and specific outcomes.	This is a valid point, but we used fairly exhaustive lists of terms for all of these vague constructs, which may be unclear in the main part of the text (though can be seen in our appendices with search terms). We will add some discussion about this.
5. Please provide any recommendations on how this report can be revised to more directly address or assist implementation needs.	
You might consider creating as appendices short checklists or worksheets, designed for use by hospital administrators, safety professionals, and worker teams to help them a) identify working conditions that can adversely impact both employee health and quality/safety of patient care and b) develop interventions to improve those conditions. This is a step beyond standard hazard evaluations, because it would flag conditions most strongly associated with patient outcomes. Many of these would be work organization domains that hazard evaluations do not normally address. These worksheets would help drive hospital interventions to address systems-level problems	We have forwarded your suggestion to the topic nominator. .
This is valuable work as it relates to the healthcare personnel it represents in the clinic setting. Such work is also needed in the acute care settings. Given that the majority of the healthcare workforce is comprised of nurses in acute care settings, I would hope that a similar review would be conducted for acute care and include nurses as part of the population of interest. Studies related to nursing impact are being done but a systematic review has not been conducted and might be valuable as healthcare strives to become more effective with delivery of services and improvement in outcomes.	Thank you. Additional topics (such as acute care settings) can be nominated at the VA ESP Web site: http://www.hsrd.research.va.gov/publications/esp/
I can't help but wonder if other important studies evaluating effect and impact of PCMH have been inadvertently excluded here because did not specifically include the three categories mentioned above.	The evidence group at the Minneapolis VA has reviewed the literature on PCMH for another VA program. To our knowledge there are no additional published reports of PCMH interventions.

APPENDIX D. EVIDENCE TABLES

Appendix D, Table 1. Description of Human Resources Practices Studies – United States

Study Country Funding Source	Sample		Study design	Working Conditions Studied[b]	Patient/Provider Outcomes Studied[c]	Study Quality[d]
	Patients[a]	Providers/Clinics				
Castro 2009[37] US *Not Reported*	Convenience sample of 218 Latina patients **Sample** Male: 0% Race/Ethnicity: 86% Mexican Age: 43% 25-32 years	Convenience sample of 15 licensed NPs from 11 urban clinics	Cross-sectional	ii. Training	v. Patient Satisfaction with Provider	1/4
DesRoches 2008[55] US *Robert Wood Johnson Foundation*	N/A	2,758 MDs (62% response rate) from the 2007 AMA file	Cross-sectional	vi. Electronic Medical Records	i. Quality of Care iv. Medication Errors	3/4
Fairchild 2001[51] Boston area *Not Reported*	**Sample** NR	132 MDs with at least 100 months working in hospital affiliated practices in urban area	Cross-sectional	iv. Hours	i. Quality of Care v. Patient Satisfaction with Provider	2/4
Feldstein 2010[56] US – WA/OR *Kaiser Permanente*	Approximately 1,500 diabetes and CVD patients from 2005-2007 **Sample** Male: NR Race/Ethnicity: 7-12 % nonwhite Age (years): 61 (diabetes), 70 (CVD)	15 Kaiser Permanente clinics: 167 PCPs with at least 20 diabetes patients 143 PCPs with at least 20 CVD patients	Retrospective cohort	vi. Electronic Medical Records	i. Quality of Care	4/4
Haas 2006[40] Utah *Health Studies Fund of the Department of Family & Preventive Medicine*	623 patients **Sample** Male: ~30% Race/Ethnicity: NR Age: 52 % 18-50 years	54 MDs and PAs at 7 urban community clinics	Pre-post of repeated cross-sections	i. Training	v. Patient Satisfaction with Provider	3/5

48

The Effect of Working Conditions on Patient Care: A Systematic Review

Study Country *Funding Source*	Sample		Study design	Working Conditions Studied[b]	Patient/Provider Outcomes Studied[c]	Study Quality[d]
	Patients[a]	Providers/Clinics				
Linzer 2009[6] US *Agency for Healthcare Research and Quality*	1,795 patients <u>Sample</u> Male: 31% Race/Ethnicity: 62% White, 22% Black Age (years): 60	119 clinics in 5 regions (urban & rural): 218 general internists and 204 family practitioners	Cross-sectional	iii. Workload v. Autonomy	i. Quality of Care iii. Non-medication Treatment Errors	3/4
Mundinger 2000[35] US *Division of Nursing, Health Resources and Services Administration, US Department of Health and Human Services; The Fan Fox and Leslie R. Samuels Foundation; and the New York State Department of Health*	1,316 patients <u>Sample</u> Male: 25% Race/Ethnicity: 1% White, 9% Black, 85% Hispanic Age (years): 44	5 urban clinics	Randomized trial	i. Skills	v. Patient Satisfaction with Provider	Allocation concealment: No Blinding: Providers were blinded Intention to treat analysis: No Withdrawals adequately described: Yes
Nyweide 2009[49] US *The Commonwealth Fund, National Institute on Aging*	N/A	71,980 PCPs with at least 10 Medicare patients (using Medicare data)	Cross-sectional	iv. Workload	i. Quality of Care	2/4
Parkerton 2003[53] US *Private (BCBS Michigan); Public (Rackam Graduate School; Dept of Health Management and policy U of Michigan)*	N/A	194 family practitioners and general internists from 25 out-patient clinics of a single medical group in western Washington	Cross-sectional	iv. Hours	i. Quality of Care v. Patient Satisfaction with Provider	3/4
Roblin 2004[36] Georgia, USA *Garland Memorial Fund of Kaiser Permanente Medical Care Program*	26,237 Kaiser Permanente Georgia patients (60% response rate) <u>Sample</u> Male: 39% Race/Ethnicity: NR Age: 76% 18-54 years	139 MDs, 63 PA/NPs	Cross-sectional	i. Skills	v. Patient Satisfaction with Provider	4/4

The Effect of Working Conditions on Patient Care: A Systematic Review

Study Country *Funding Source*	Sample		Study design	Working Conditions Studied[b]	Patient/Provider Outcomes Studied[c]	Study Quality[d]
	Patients[a]	Providers/Clinics				
Weiner 2009[57] US *National Institute on Aging*	40,487 referrals **Sample** Male: 33% Race/Ethnicity: 54% non-white Age: 20% 21-39 years	10 PC clinics	Pre-post of repeated cross-sections	vi. Electronic Medical Records	i. Quality of Care	5/5
Zabar 2010[41] US *Public: NYU Student Health Center*	**Sample** NR	21 NYU Student Health Center clinicians (14 MDs, 6 NPs, 1 PA)	Pre-post	ii. Training	i. Quality of Care v. Patient Satisfaction with Provider	4/5

Notes: a. To the extent possible, we report the following descriptive statistics (means/percents) on the main patient sample analyzed: age, gender, race, and veteran status. "NR" means this information was not reported in the study and "N/A" means the statistics were not applicable to the sample studied.

b. We focus on the following human resources practices, noting that each construct may be measured differently across studies:

i. Skills
ii. Training
iii. Workload
iv. Hours/Scheduling
v. Autonomy
vi. Electronic Medical Records or Computerized Systems

c. We focus on the following patient and provider outcomes (vii-viii), noting that each construct may be measured differently across studies:

i. Quality of Care – Clinical Effectiveness or Access
ii. Patient Safety- Diagnostic Errors
iii. Patient Safety – Non-Medication Treatment Errors
iv. Patient Safety – Medication Treatment Errors
v. Patient Satisfaction with Provider
vi. Patient Satisfaction with Clinic/Care
vii. Provider Stress
viii. Provider Satisfaction

d. We assessed study quality in the following ways. For non-randomized studies, we assessed the risk of study bias on the following dimensions: population (e.g., representative, uniform inclusion/exclusion criteria), outcomes (important outcomes assessed and measured, appropriate follow-up), measurement (variables uniformly assessed, blinded, construct valid measures), confounding (design and methods minimize confounding) and whether the intervention can be replicated if applicable. Study quality for these studies is reported as the number of criteria met (where risk was assessed as low) out of the total possible dimensions evaluated for risk. For randomized studies, we assessed study quality based on the four criteria listed.

Abbreviations used: AMA = American Medical Association, CVD = cardiovascular disease, GP = general practitioner, MD = physician, N/A = not applicable, NP = Nurse practitioner, NR = not reported, PA = Physician Assistant, PC = primary care, PCP = primary care provider

The Effect of Working Conditions on Patient Care: A Systematic Review

Appendix D, Table 2. Description of Human Resources Practices Studies – Europe

Study Country *Funding Source*	Sample		Study design	Working Conditions Studied[b]	Patient/Provider Outcomes Studied[c]	Study Quality[d]
	Patients[a]	Providers/Clinics				
Caldow 2006[32] Scotland *Chief Scientist Office, Department of Health, Scottish Executive*	1,343 randomly selected patients (49% response rate) **Sample** Male: 41% Race: NR Age: 41% 16-44 years	22 practices (55% response rate) in mostly urban areas	Cross-sectional	i. Skills	v. Patient Satisfaction with Provider vi. Patient Satisfaction with Practice/Care	2/4
Campbell 2001[42] England *National Primary Care Research and Development Centre*	4,493 patients (38% response rate) **Sample** NR	60 randomly selected practices across 6 districts in England (80% response rate)	Retrospective cohort	iii. Workload	i. Quality of Care	1/4
Campbell 2005[43] London *North Thames Region of the NHS Executive*	7,247 patients (66% response rate) **Sample** NR	54 volunteer practices (27% response rate) in urban areas	Cross-sectional	iii. Workload	i. Quality of Care	2/4
Carlsen 2006[44] Norway *Research Council of Norway through the Programme for Health Economics*	829 patients **Sample** Male: 29% Race: NR Age (years): 49	41 GPs (23% response rate)	Cross-sectional	iii. Workload	v. Patient Satisfaction with Provider	3/4
Dierick-van Daele 2009[33] Netherlands *Dutch Ministry of Health, Welfare and Sport and the Health Insurances CZ and VGZ, Foundation ROS Robuust, The Province of North-Brabant, the Netherlands*	1,397 patients **Sample** Male: 39% Race: NR Age: 52 % 16 to 45 years	Convenience sample of 12 NPs and 50 GPs in 15 clinics	Randomized controlled trial	i. Skills	vi. Patient Satisfaction with Provider	Allocation concealment: Yes Blinding: No (reported to be impossible for this study) Intention to treat analysis: No Withdrawals adequately described: Yes

The Effect of Working Conditions on Patient Care: A Systematic Review

Study Country Funding Source	Sample Patients[a]	Providers/Clinics	Study design	Working Conditions Studied[b]	Patient/Provider Outcomes Studied[c]	Study Quality[d]
Edwards 2004[38] South Wales Department of Health, Health in Partnership Programme	747 patients (44% response rate) Sample NR	20 GPs (41% response rate)	Cluster randomized crossover trial	ii. Training	v. Patient Satisfaction with Provider	Allocation concealment: Yes Blinding: Yes (assessors of clinic visits) Intention to treat analysis: No Withdrawals adequately described: No
French 2001[52] UK Medical Research Council	661 patients (66% response rate) Sample NR	26 GPs in England	Longitudinal (cohort of GPs, repeated cross-sections of patients)	iv. Hours	v. Patient Satisfaction with Provider vi. Patient Satisfaction with Practice/Care	1/4
Grytten 2009[46] Norway Not reported	1,920 patients Sample Male: 46% Race: NR Age: 51% 16 to 45 years	1,075 GPs	Cross-sectional	iii. Workload	vi. Patient Satisfaction with Practice/Care	4/4
Laurant 2007[34] Netherlands Private	117 patients (50% response rate) Sample Male: 40% Race: NR Age (years): 63.9	30 GPs, 5 NPs, in 20 clinics	Cross-sectional	i. Skills	v. Patient Satisfaction with Provider	2/4
Luras 2007[47] Norway Research Council of Norway	2,326 patients Sample Male: 42% Race: NR Age: 47% 16 to 45 years	NR	Cross-sectional	iii. Workload	v. Patient Satisfaction with Provider	4/4

Study Country Funding Source	Sample		Study design	Working Conditions Studied[b]	Patient/Provider Outcomes Studied[c]	Study Quality[d]
	Patients[a]	Providers/Clinics				
Magan 2011[48] Madrid, Spain *Spanish Ministry of Health*	102,346 hospitalizations of adults age 65+ **Sample** Male: NR Race: NR Age (years): 77 for men, 81 for women	34 health districts in Madrid	Cross-sectional ecological	iii. Workload	i. Quality of Care	4/4
McKinstry 2007[54] Scotland *Not Reported*	**Sample stats NR**	276 MDs (62% response rate) with at least 49 patient surveys each	Cross-sectional	v. Autonomy	vi. Patient Satisfaction with Practice/Care	1/4
Salisbury 2010[50] UK *NHS Research and Development Programme on Service and Delivery Organisation*	4,573 patients (84% response rate) **Sample** Male: 39% Race: 98% white Age (years): 52	150 GPs in 27 practices in England	Cross-sectional	iii. Workload	v. Patient Satisfaction with Provider vi. Patient Satisfaction with Practice/Care	4/4

Notes: See notes from Appendix D, Table 1

Appendix D, Table 3. Description of Human Resources Practices Studies – Outside of US or Europe

Study Country Funding Source	Sample		Study design	Working Conditions Studied[b]	Patient/Provider Outcomes Studied[c]	Study Quality[d]
	Patients[a]	Providers/Clinics				
Dong 2010[45] China *Public (Chinese Ministry of Health (MOH) the United Nations Children's Fund (Unicef)*	20,125 prescriptions **Sample** Male: 57% Race: NR; Age (years): 34	680 primary health clinics from 40 rural counties	Cross-sectional	iii. Workload	iv. Medication Errors	4/4
Goulet 2007[39] Canada *Not Reported*	N/A	51 MDs who participated in a remedial professional development program (RPDP)	Pre-post	ii. Training	i. Quality of Care	3/5

Notes: See notes from Appendix D, Table 1

Appendix D, Table 4. Quality of Care Outcomes - Human Resources Practices Studies

First Author, Year	HR Practice & Measure[a]	Access		Effectiveness	
		Measured as:	Main Finding	Measured as:	Main Finding
US STUDIES					
DesRoches 2008[55]	vi. EMR: a)"Full" System – gives warnings, reminders for guideline based care, ability to order tests vs. b)"Basic" System – no order entry capability or clinical decision support	NR	NR	Physician response to: has the EMR ever helped to: a) alert to critical lab value b) provide preventive care c) order a critical laboratory test d) order a genetic test	a) 90% in full system vs. 75% in basic system; (p=0.004) b) 69% in full system vs. 41% in basic system (p<0.001) c) 68% in full system vs. 36 in basic system. (p<0.001) d) 17% in full system vs. 8% in basic system (p=0.03)
Fairchild 2001[51]	iv. Hours- Part time (PT) vs. Full time (FT)	NR	NR	Compliant with quality measure: whether 70% of patients had appropriate screening for Pap smear, mammography, and cholesterol	80% of PT PCPs versus 75% of FT PCPs were compliant (p-value = 0.04)
Feldstein 2010[56]	vi. EMR–electronic tool that identifies care gaps for each patient	NR	NR	"Care score" based on % of care recommendations met by PCPs per member month (out of 100)	After implementation, diabetes care score increased by 7.64 (p<0.001) and CVD care score increased by 5.10 (p<0.001)
Linzer 2009[6]	iii. Workload – time needed per patient/per allotted; chaotic office (0/1) v. Autonomy – work control 14 item scale (0/1)	NR	NR	3 quality indices based on management of 3 chronic conditions: a) hypertension b) diabetes c) heart failure	Greater time pressure yielded slightly lower quality. A chaotic office had no effect on quality. Having greater work control resulted in greater quality.
Nyweide 2009[49]	iii. Workload – Medicare caseload	NR	NR	a) % of appropriate women who get mammograms b) % of diabetics who receive hemoglobin A1c test c) preventable hospitalization rate	Providers with at least a) 328 women, b) 438 diabetics, and c) 19,069 patients are needed to detect a 10% difference in quality of care of Medicare patients relative to the national mean
Parkerton 2003[53]	iv. Hours- continuous measure of MD appointment hours (3 to 35 hours)	NR	NR	a) % of patients receiving cancer (Pap smear and mammography) screening b) % of patients receiving recommended diabetes care	a) Cancer screening coefficient: -0.07 (p=0.01) b) Diabetes management coefficient= -0.11 (p=0.008)
Weiner 2009[57]	vi. EMR – electronic referrals	Getting a specialty appointment scheduled from a referral (0/1)	OR of getting a specialty appointment scheduled increased by 4.32 (p <0.001) after implementation	NR	

54

The Effect of Working Conditions on Patient Care: A Systematic Review

First Author, Year	HR Practice & Measure[a]	Access		Effectiveness	
		Measured as:	Main Finding	Measured as:	Main Finding
Zabar 2010[41]	ii. Training -communication skills workshops	NR	NR	Chart Audits for documented risk screenings of: a) smoking b) depressed mood c) anhedonia d) sexual activity e) drinking alcohol	Mantel-Haenszel RRs: a) 1.65 (p=0.03) b) 1.40 (p=0.04) c) 1.47 (p=0.01) d) 1.73 (p=0.002) e) 1.77 (p=0.04)
EUROPEAN STUDIES					
Cambell 2001[42]	iii. Workload -booking interval (amount of time between each appointment)			Score based on guideline concordant care for three conditions: a) adult asthma b) angina c) type 2 diabetes mellitus	Mean unadjusted differences between scores of practices with 10+ intervals between appointments and those with 5 minute intervals: a) adult asthma – 21.6 (p <0.001) b) angina – 10.2 (p=0.002) c) type 2 diabetes – 10 (p=0.028)
Campbell 2005[43]	iii. Workload -list size	Two measures created based on patient report of how quickly usually seen after appointment request: a) See doctor the same or next day (0/1) b) See doctor within 2-3 days (0/1)	Correlations: a) -0.37(p=0.007) b) -0.21 (p=0.133)		
Magan 2011[48]	iii. Workload -visits/day	NR	NR	Rate of Ambulatory Care Sensitive Hospitalizations (ACSH)	Each additional patient per workday was associated with 6% to 7% higher relative rate of ACSH (p<0.001)
STUDIES OUTSIDE THE US & EUROPE					
Goulet 2007[39]	ii. Training – participation in a remedial professional development program			Expert physician peer review of medical records on: a) clinical investigation b) diagnostic accuracy c) treatment and follow-up	a) 46% of providers improved in clinical investigation (p<0.001) b) 29% improved in diagnostic accuracy (p=0.01) and c) 36% improved in treatment and follow-up (p<0.001)

Notes: a. We focus on the following human resources practices:
  i.   Skills
  ii. Training
  iii. Workload
  iv. Hours/Scheduling
  v.   Autonomy
  vi. Electronic Medical Records or Computerized Systems

Abbreviations used: CVD= cardiovascular disease, EMR = electronic medical record, GP = general practitioner, MD = physician, NP = nurse practitioner, NR = not reported, NS = not statistically significant, OR = odds ratio, PA = physician assistant, PCP = primary care provider, RR = relative risk

Appendix D, Table 5. Patient Safety Outcomes – Human Resources Practices Studies

First Author, Year	HR Practice & Measure[a]	Diagnostic Errors		Non-Medication Treatment Errors		Medication Errors	
		Measured as:	Main Finding	Measured as:	Main Finding	Measured as:	Main Finding
US STUDIES							
DesRoches 2008[55]	vi. EMRs: a) Full System—gives warnings, reminders for guideline based care, ability to order tests vs. b) Basic System – no order entry capability or clinical decision support	NR	NR	NR	NR	Physician report of whether EMR ever helped: 1) prevent drug allergy 2) prevent dangerous medication interaction	1) 80 vs. 66% of MDs in full vs. basic report system helped with drug allergies (p=0.01) 2) 71 vs. 54% of MDs in full vs. basic report system prevented dangerous interactions (p=0.002)
Linzer 2009[6]	iii. Workload: a) time needed/patient/per allotted b) chaotic office (0/1) v. Autonomy a) work control 14 item scale (0/1)	NR	NR	Score based on chart audits to gauge missed treatment opportunities, inattention to behavioral factors, and guideline nonadherence (0/100)	No significant effect of workload on prevention, hypertension or diabetes management errors. Having more autonomy resulted in a lower total error score (more errors) (coefficient = -2.80, (-5.72, 0.12).	NR	NR
STUDIES OUTSIDE THE US & EUROPE							
Dong 2010[45]	iii. Workload -patient visits/month	NR	NR	NR	NR	Polypharmacy (Rx's with 5 or more drugs) per 100 patient-visits/month (0/1)	OR of Polypharmacy w/ higher workload versus less workload = 1.70 [1.26, 2.29]

Notes: a. We focus on the following human resources practices:

vii.   Skills
viii.   Training
ix.   Workload
x.   Hours/Scheduling
xi.   Autonomy
xii.   Electronic Medical Records or Computerized Systems

Abbreviations used: CVD= cardiovascular disease, EMR = electronic medical record, GP = general practitioner, MD = physician, NP = nurse practitioner, NR = not reported, NS = not statistically significant, OR = odds ratio, PA = physician assistant, PCP = primary care provider, RR = relative risk

Appendix D, Table 6. Patient Satisfaction Outcomes – Human Resources Practices Studies

First Author, Year	HR Practice & Measure	Patient Satisfaction with Provider		Patient Satisfaction with Practice or Care	
		Measured as:	Main Finding	Measured as:	Main Finding
US STUDIES					
Castro 2009[37]	ii. Training -NP reported receipt of cultural competence training	Patient Satisfaction Questionnaire (PSQ-III)	Patient satisfaction positively correlated with NP's culture competence training (r=0.32, p-value=NR)	NR	NR
Fairchild 2001[51]	iv. Hours– Part time (PT) vs. Full time (FT)	% of patients surveyed rating PCP as "excellent" or "good"	FT = 92%, PT = 95% (p=0.13)	NR	NR
Haas 2006[40]	ii. Training -90 minute workshop on structuring visits effectively	Patient reported satisfaction scaled from 1 (better) to 5 (worse) based on 30 items	Overall satisfaction: Pre-test= 1.12 Post-test = 1.14 (p = NS)	NR	NR
Mundinger 2000[35]	i. Skills -visit with MD -visit with NP	Satisfaction mean score measured by a 15 item satisfaction survey (5-point scale)	Overall Satisfaction Baseline: MD =4.6; NP = 4.59 (p= 0.89) 6 month F/U: MD = 4.46; NP = 4.45 (p=0.87)	NR	NR
Roblin 2004[36]	i. Skills - visit with GP vs. - visit with PA/NP	Practitioner interaction (5 items)	1.16 (p<0.05) times more likely to be satisfied with practitioner interaction when seeing a PA/NP vs. an MD	Care access (4 items)	No significant difference satisfaction with care access whether patient saw an MD vs. PA/NP
Parkerton 2003[53]	iv. Hours- continuous measure of MD appointment hours (3 to 35 hours)	Patient satisfaction = excellent	Coefficient: -0.05 (p=0.21)	NR	NR
Zabar 2010[41]	ii. Training -communication skills workshops	10 point item on satisfaction with patient-provider communication[1]	No change in patient satisfaction after training		
EUROPEAN STUDIES					
Caldow 2006[32]	i. Skills - visit with GP vs. - visit with NP	NR	NR	Survey question on satisfaction with last visit dichotomized to be equal to one if patient reports "excellent" or "very good" satisfaction and 0, otherwise	No significant difference in satisfaction except patients who saw a NP were more satisfied with the amount of time spent with provider than those who saw a GP (p<0.05)

The Effect of Working Conditions on Patient Care: A Systematic Review

First Author, Year	HR Practice & Measure	Patient Satisfaction with Provider		Patient Satisfaction with Practice or Care	
		Measured as:	Main Finding	Measured as:	Main Finding
Carlsen 2006[44]	iii. Workload -GP listsize/1000	6 point survey question on how satisfied with doctor you visited dichotomized to be equal to one if patient reports "very satisfied" and 0, otherwise	No significant effect of GP listsize on patient satisfaction	NR	NR
Dierick-van Daele 2009[33]	i. Skills - visit with GP vs. - visit with NP	10 point scale (details not reported) on overall patient satisfaction	No significant difference in patient satisfaction across GP vs. NP patients (p=0.83)	NR	NR
Edwards 2004[38]	ii. Training - Shared decision making (SDM) - Risk communication (RC)	Patient satisfaction with the decision made (single item)	No significant effect of either training on satisfaction: SDM coefficient = 0.1 (p=NS) RC coefficient = 0.5 (p=NS)	NR	NR
French 2001[52]	iv. Hours -GPs being "on call" or off duty	General Satisfaction subscale on Consultant Satisfaction Score (CSQ)	Visits surrounding "On call" = 75.6 Visits surrounding "Off duty" 77.1 (p=NS)	Professional Care subscale on CSQ	Visits surrounding "on call" =75.3 Visits surrounding "Off duty" =76.8 (p=NS)
Grytten 2009[46]	iii. Workload - # of consultations per person on the GP's list	NR	NR	Patient response to a) how satisfied with wait time to get an appointment (4 point scale) b) satisfaction with amount of time the GP spent (4 point scale)	Probit coefficients: a) 0.938 (p < 0.05) b) 0.055 (p=0.13)
Laurant 2007[34]	i. Skills - visit with GP vs. - visit with NP	Overall satisfaction using the "Chronically ill patients evaluate general practice" scale (6 point scale)	Satisfaction with: a) GP = 4.1 b) NP = 4.4 (p = 0.03)	NR	NR
Luras 2007[47]	iii. Workload -listsize longer than stated -listsize shorter than stated	Satisfaction (5 point scales) with a) doctor taking questions/ problems seriously b) getting a referral c) length of time with doctor	Longer listsize than stated adjusted ORs: a) 2.0 [0.84, 4.75] b) 1.03 [0.68, 1.57] c) 0.84 [0.62, 1.16] Shorter listsize than stated adjusted ORs: a) 0.41 [0.23,0.72] b) 0.48 [0.33,0.72] c) 0.63 [0.44, 0.92]	Satisfaction (5 point scales) with a) confidence in treatment prescribed b) waiting time	Longer listsize than stated adjusted ORs: a) 2.17 [0.98,4.82] b) 0.66 [0.51, 0.84] Shorter listsize than stated adjusted ORs: a) 0.46 [0.27, 0.78] b) 1.67 [1.17, 2.39]
McKinstry 2007[54]	vi. Autonomy -control of work on the Morale Assessment in General Practice Index	NR	NR	Patient rating of a) how treated by receptionists b) length of time you have to wait (higher is better)	Correlations (r): a) -0.15 (p=0.02) b) -0.21 (p<0.01)

First Author, Year	HR Practice & Measure	Patient Satisfaction with Provider		Patient Satisfaction with Practice or Care	
		Measured as:	Main Finding	Measured as:	Main Finding
Salisbury 2010[50]	iv. Workload -listsize (per 1000 patients)	Overall satisfaction (7 point scale)	Coefficient = 0.01 (p=0.32)	Satisfaction with: a) ability to get an appointment (6 point scale) b) access (0 to 100 scale created from 6 questions about contacting practice, making an appointment)	Coefficients a) 0.13 (p=0.001) b) 0.68 (p=0.25)

Notes: a. We focus on the following human resources practices:
i.   Skills
ii. Training
iii. Workload
iv. Hours/Scheduling
v.   Autonomy
vi. Electronic Medical Records or Computerized Systems

Abbreviations used: CVD= cardiovascular disease, GP = general practitioner, MD = physician, NP = nurse practitioner, NR = not reported, NS = not statistically significant, OR = odds ratio, PA = physician assistant, PCP = primary care provider, RR = relative risk

Appendix D, Table 7. Description of Organizational Culture Studies

Study Country Funding Source	Sample		Study design	Working Conditions Studied	Patient/ Provider Outcomes Studied	Study Quality
	Patients	Providers/Clinics				
Adam 2010[65] US Not Reported	N=20 Intervention (n=12) Control (n=8) **Sample** Male: 35% Race: 70% white, 35% black Median age (years): Team care = 49, Usual care = 50	NR	Case-control	vii. Team-based care	ii. Quality of Care -Effectiveness vii. Patient Satisfaction with Care	0/5

The Effect of Working Conditions on Patient Care: A Systematic Review

Study Country *Funding Source*	Sample		Study design	Working Conditions Studied	Patient/ Provider Outcomes Studied	Study Quality
	Patients	Providers/Clinics				
Bean-Mayberry 2003[62] US *Department of Veterans Affairs*	n=971 female veterans (62% of respondents were from women's clinics, 38% from traditional primary care) **Sample** Male: 0% Race: 87% white, 10% black, 3% other Veteran (%): 100 Age (years): 58.3	8 Veterans Affairs Medical Centers in 3 states	Cross-sectional (survey)	ix. Care environment (women's clinic vs. traditional primary care clinic)	vii. Patient Satisfaction with Care	1/5
Boyd 2009[66] US *John A. Hartford Foundation, Agency for Healthcare Research and Quality, National Institute for Aging, Jacob & Valeria Langeloth Foundation, Kaiser-Permanente Mid-Atlantic States, Johns Hopkins HealthCare, Roger C. Lipitz Center for Integrated Health Care*	N=904 **Sample** Male: 45.2% Race: 50% white. 46% African American, 4% other Age (years): 77.6	NR	Cluster-randomized controlled trial	vii. Team-based care	vii. Patient Satisfaction with Care	Allocation concealment: No Blinding: No Intention to treat analysis (ITT): Yes Withdrawals/ dropouts adequately described: Yes
Chomienne 2011[67] Canada Not Reported	N= 319 provided baseline data 376 received psych services **Sample** Male: 30% Age (years): 83.6% (over 25) Race: 94% White, 6% Other Insurance Coverage for psych services: 43.8% No, 32.3% Yes, 23.9% Don't Know Clinic Location: 43% Rural, 57% urban	N/A	Prospective cohort	vii. Team-based care	Patient: ii. Quality of Care - Effectiveness Provider: Physician satisfaction	1/5

Study Country *Funding Source*	Sample		Study design	Working Conditions Studied	Patient/ Provider Outcomes Studied	Study Quality
	Patients	Providers/Clinics				
Gilfillan 2010[63] US *Not Reported*	N= 15,310 <u>Sample</u> Male: 49.7% Age (years): 73.8 Admissions/1000 members/ year: 283.6 Readmissions/ 1000/year: 46	NR	Pre-post	viii. PCMH	ii. Quality of Care - Effectiveness	2/5
Hogg 2009[68] Canada *Ontario Ministry of Health and LongTerm Care Transition Fund*	N=241 <u>Sample</u> Male: 35.3% Age (years): 71.2	NR	Randomized controlled trial	vii. Team-based care	ii. Quality of Care - Effectiveness	Allocation concealment: No Blinding: Yes Intention to treat analysis (ITT): Yes Withdrawals/ dropouts adequately described: Yes
Linzer 2009[6] US *Agency for Healthcare Research and Quality*	N= 1,795 <u>Sample</u> Male: 31% Race/Ethnicity: 62% White, 22% Black Age (years): 60	119 clinics in 5 regions (urban & rural) 218 general internists and 204 family practitioners	Cross-sectional	x. Clinic values	ii. Quality of Care - Effectiveness	3/4
Reid 2009[64] US *Group Health Cooperative*	N= 236,604 PCMH clinic (n=8,094) 19 Control clinics (n=228,510) <u>Sample</u> Group visit attendance (%): 0.02 Attended self-management support workshops (%): 0.02 Health risk assessment completion (%): 1.8 Pre-visit outreach (%): 1.1 Emergency/urgent care follow-up (%): 6.5	N= 82 83% Response rate <u>Sample</u> Male: 16.3%	Prospective pre-post	viii. PCMH	<u>Patient:</u> ii. Quality of Care - Effectiveness vi. Patient Satisfaction with Provider vii. Patient Satisfaction with Care <u>Provider:</u> Staff Burnout	2/5

The Effect of Working Conditions on Patient Care: A Systematic Review

Study Country Funding Source	Sample		Study design	Working Conditions Studied	Patient/ Provider Outcomes Studied	Study Quality
	Patients	Providers/Clinics				
Sellors 2003[69] Canada *Health Transition Fund, Health Canada, the Department of Family Medicine, McMaster University, and the Centre for Evaluation of Medicines, St. Joseph's Healthcare, Hamilton, Ont*	N=889 **Sample** Male: 37.2% Race: NR Age (years): 74 Mean length of time with physician: 10.9 years Intervention (Pharmacist consult): n=431 Usual Care: n=458	N=48 agreed to participate Age: NR Male: 67% Race: NR Years since graduation: 21.7 Intervention (Pharmacist consult): n=24 Usual Care: n=24	Randomized controlled trial	vii. Team-based care	v. Medication Errors	Allocation concealment: No Blinding: No Intention to treat analysis (ITT): No Withdrawals/ dropouts adequately described: Yes

Notes: a. To the extent possible, we report the following descriptive statistics (means/percents) on the main patient sample analyzed: age, gender, race, and veteran status. "NR" means this information was not reported in the study and "N/A" means the statistics were not applicable to the sample studied.

b. We focus on the following organizational culture components:

   vii.   Team-based Care

   viii. Patient Centered Medical Home (PCMH)

   ix.   Care Environment

   x.   Clinic Values

c. We focus on the following patient and provider outcomes (vii-viii), noting that each construct may be measured differently across studies:

   i.   Quality of Care – Clinical Effectiveness or Access

   ii.   Patient Safety- Diagnostic Errors

   iii.   Patient Safety – Non-Medication Treatment Errors

   iv.   Patient Safety – Medication Treatment Errors

   v.   Patient Satisfaction with Provider

   vi.   Patient Satisfaction with Clinic/Care

   vii.   Provider Stress

   viii. Provider Satisfaction

d. We assessed study quality in the following ways. For non-randomized studies, we assessed the risk of study bias on the following dimensions: population (e.g., representative, uniform inclusion/exclusion criteria), outcomes (important outcomes assessed and measured, appropriate follow-up), measurement (variables uniformly assessed, blinded, construct valid measures), confounding (design and methods minimize confounding) and whether the intervention can be replicated if applicable. Study quality for these studies is reported as the number of criteria met (where risk was assessed as low) out of the total possible dimensions evaluated for risk. For randomized studies, we assessed study quality based on the four criteria listed.

Abbreviations used: GP = general practitioner, MD = physician, N/A = not applicable, NP = Nurse practitioner, NR = not reported, PA = Physician Assistant, PC = primary care, PCMH = patient centered medical home, PCP = primary care provider

The Effect of Working Conditions on Patient Care: A Systematic Review

Appendix D, Table 8. Quality of Care Outcomes – Organizational Culture Studies

Study	Organizational Culture Practice & Measure	Access		Effectiveness	
		Measured as:	Main Finding	Measured as:	Main Finding
Adam 2010[65]	vii. Team-based Care – care team consisting of weekly team (physician, nurses, and front desk staff)	NR	NR	Median # of Hospitalizations and ER visits	Hospitalizations: Team Care (n=12): Baseline = 0, 6 month = 0; Usual Care (n=8): Baseline = 0, 6 month = 0; ER visits – Team Care (n=12): 6 months before = 0, 6 month = 0.5; Usual Care (n=8): 6 months before = 0.5, 6 month = 0.5
Chomienne 2011[67]	vii. Team-based Care – addition of a psychologist to family practice clinic	NR	NR	- Outcome Questionnaire 45 (OQ-45) – standardized symptom distress inventory -EuroQoL(EQ-5D) - and index of health-related quality of life	OQ-45 improved in 60% of patients; EQ-5D (quality of life) improved for 83% of patients who completed first and last assessment (n=178; p<0.001)
Gilfillan 2010[63]	viii. PCMH- multi-component intervention	NR	NR	Admissions (members/year) Readmissions (members/year)	Admissions: PCMH = 257 admissions/ 1000 members/ year; -18% [95% CI -30% to -5%; P<0.01]; Control= 313 admissions/ 1000 members/ year[§]; Readmission: PCMH= 38/1000 members/year; -36% [95% CI, -55 to -3%; p=0.02]; Control= 59/1000 members/year[§]
Hogg 2009[68]	vii. Team-based care – Anticipatory and Preventive Team Care (APTCare) consisting of physicians, 1-3 nurse practitioners, and a pharmacist			A Chronic Disease Management (CDM) Quality of Care (QOC) composite score based on 12 indicator processes for 4 chronic diseases (CAD, diabetes, CHF, and COPD)	CDM QOC +9.29%; [p<0.001] Preventive Care +16.5%; [P<0.001]

The Effect of Working Conditions on Patient Care: A Systematic Review

Study	Organizational Culture Practice & Measure	Access		Effectiveness	
		Measured as:	Main Finding	Measured as:	Main Finding
Linzer 2009[6]	x. Clinic values	NR	NR	Association of clinic values and total quality based on management of: a) hypertension b) diabetes, and c) Preventive care from medical record audits.	Quality emphasis 0.94 (4.07 to 5.95) Information and communication emphasis 4.65 (0.07 to 9.23) Trust in organization 1.88 (2.97 to 6.73) Workplace cohesiveness 0.85 (3.37 to 5.07) Values alignment 1.15 (3.47 to 5.78)
Reid 2009[64]	viii. PCMH multi-component intervention	NR	NR	Contacts/ 1000 members/ year	Admissions (ACSC): PCMH= 12/1000; RR=0.89; P<0.001 Usual Care= 13/1000 members/year Admissions: PCMH=100/1000 members/year RR=1.03 (NS) Usual Care= 100/1000 members/year

Notes: We focus on the following organizational culture components:
  i.   Team-based Care
  ii.   Patient Centered Medical Home (PCMH)
  iii. Care Environment
  iv.   Clinic Values

Abbreviations used: ACSC = Ambulatory Care Sensitive Conditions, BP = blood pressure, CAD = coronary artery disease, CHF = congestive heart failure, COPD = chronic obstructive pulmonary disease, ER = emergency room, LDL = low density lipoprotein, LEAP = lower extremity amputation prevention, NS = not statistically significant, PCMH = patient centered medical home, QOC = quality of care

§ Controls are for simulated non-PCMH participants representing the expected outcomes from the active group if the PCMH had never been implemented

Appendix D, Table 9. Patient Safety Outcomes – Organizational Culture Studies

Author, Year	Organizational Culture Practice & Measure	Diagnostic Errors		Non-Medication Treatment Errors		Medication Errors	
		Measured as:	Main Finding	Measured as:	Main Finding	Measured as:	Main Finding
Sellors 2003[69]	vii. Team-based care -Pharmacist consultation with family physician	NR	NR	NR	NR	At least 1 drug related problem identified by the pharmacist	344/431 (79.8%) 2.5 drug related problems/ senior *No comparison data from non pharmacist control

Abbreviations used: NR = not reported

Appendix D, Table 10. Patient Satisfaction Outcomes – Organizational Culture Studies

Author, Year	Organizational Culture Practice & Measure	Patient Satisfaction with Provider		Patient Satisfaction with Practice or Care	
		Measured as:	Main Finding	Measured as:	Main Finding
Adam 2010[65]	vii. Team-based Care – care team consisting of weekly team physician, nurses, and front desk staff)	NR	NR	Patient Self-rated well-being Patient Satisfaction	<u>Patient self-rated well-being:</u> Team based = +8% Usual care = no change <u>Patient Satisfaction:</u> Team based = satisfied or very satisfied increased from 75% at baseline to 92% at 6 months Usual care = "All control patients were very satisfied or satisfied at baseline and follow-up
Bean-Mayberry 2003[62]	ix. Care environment (women's clinic vs. traditional primary care clinic)	NR	NR	Primary Care Satisfaction Survey for Women (PCSSW) a) Overall Satisfaction b) Getting Care c) Privacy/Comfort d) Communication e) Complete Care f) Follow-up Care	<u>Odds Ratios</u> a) OR=1.42(1.00-2.02) b) OR=1.69(1.14-2.49) c) OR=1.63(1.11-2.39) d) OR=1.66(1.16-2.37) e) OR=1.69(1.17-2.43) f) OR=1.70(1.16-2.47)
Boyd 2009[66]	vii. Team Based Care- "Guided Care" RN trained in chronic care integrated into primary care to work with 2-5 physicians	NR	NR	Patient Assessment of Chronic Illness Care (PACIC)	Compared to usual care, patients who received guided were twice as likely to rate chronic care highly (AOR=2.13 [95% CI=1.30 to 3.5 p=0.003])
Reid 2009[64]	viii. PCMH	Ambulatory Care Experiences Survey (ACES)* *Survey results from n=1,024 at PCMH clinic and n=1,662 at 2 control clinics	<u>ACES (Adjusted mean difference in scores):</u> Quality of GP-patient interactions= 2.12; p<0.01 Shared Decision Making= 2.76; p<0.01 Coordination of Care= 3.38; p<0.001 Access = 3.48; p<0.001	Patient Assessment of Chronic Illness Care (PACIC) survey* -Patient involvement in care -Degree teams helped set and refine goals	<u>PACIC (Adjusted mean difference in scores):</u> Patient Activation/Involvement= 3.30; p<0.01 Goal Setting/Tailoring= 3.10; p<0.05

Notes: We focus on the following organizational culture components:
vii. Team-based Care
viii. Patient Centered Medical Home (PCMH)
ix. Care Environment
x. Clinic Values

Abbreviations used: AOR = adjusted odds ratio, CI = confidence interval, GP = general practitioner, NR = not reported, OR = odds ratio, RN = registered nurse

Appendix D, Table 11. Provider Outcomes – Organizational Culture Studies

Study	Job Stress		Job Satisfaction		Burnout	
	Measured as:	Main Finding	Measured as:	Main Finding	Measured as:	Main Finding
Chomienne 2011[67]	NR	NR	Physician questionnaire on 5 point scale	8/10 doctors reported improved office atmosphere and quality of life at work 7/10 reported improved workload	NR	NR
Linzer 2009[6]	Association with physician rated clinic values: a) Quality emphasis: b) Information and comm. Emphasis: c) Trust in organization: d) Workplace cohesiveness: e) Values alignment:	a) -0.34 (-0.48 to -0.20) b) -0.25 (-0.37 to -0.13) c) -0.31 (-0.43 to -0.19) d) -0.25 (-0.39 to -0.11) e) -0.34 (-0.46 to -0.22)	Association with physician rated clinic values: a) Quality emphasis: b) Information and comm. Emphasis: c) Trust in organization: d) Workplace cohesiveness: e) Values alignment:	a) 0.51 (0.41 to 0.61) b) 0.32 (0.21 to 0.42) c) 0.55 (0.45 to 0.65) d) 0.43 (0.30 to 0.59) e) 0.48 (0.37 to 0.59)	Association with physician rated clinic values: a) Quality emphasis: b) Information and comm. Emphasis: c) Trust in organization: d) Workplace cohesiveness: e) Values alignment:	a) -0.57 (-0.76 to -0.37) b) -0.33 (-0.51 to -0.14) c) -0.51 (-0.69 to -0.34) d) -0.33 (-0.50 to -0.15) e) -0.49 (-0.66 to -0.33)
Reid 2009[64]	NR	NR	NR	NR	Maslach Burnout Inventory	10% of PCMH staff reported emotional exhaustion vs. 30% of control clinics p<0.01

Notes: We focus on the following organizational culture components:
   vii.   Team-based Care
   viii. Patient Centered Medical Home (PCMH)
   ix.   Care Environment
   x.   Clinic Values

Abbreviations used: NR = not reported

Appendix D, Table 12. Description of Physical Environment Studies

Study Country *Funding Source*	Sample		Study Design	Working Conditions Studied	Patient/Provider Outcomes Studied	Study Quality
	Patients	Providers/Clinics				
Arneill 2002[71] United States *None Reported*	n=147 college students Male: 27% Race: "majority Caucasian" Age: NR (range 18-24 years) Veteran (%): NR n=48 senior citizens Male: 34% Race: "primarily Caucasian" Age: NR (range 59-90 years) Veteran (%): NR	Slides of 35 waiting rooms (analyzed data from 34 slides)	Case series	Environment (waiting areas)	Perceived quality of care Comfort in environment	0/3 relevant criteria
Rice 2008[70] United Kingdom *Government*	Phase 1, n=1118 Male: 35.1 Race: NR Age (years): 48.8 Phase 2, n=954 Male: 34.8% Race: NR Age (years): 47.8 NOTE: unmatched patients (Phase 1 vs. Phase 2)	n=19 with data from Phase 1 and twice in Phase 2 (4 and 11 months after move); 13 administrative/ reception staff, 6 health professionals	Before and after Patient questionnaire completion rate 80% in both phases	Environment (lighting, sound, space, privacy, furnishings, art)	Patient anxiety, satisfaction Staff well-being, job satisfaction Patient-doctor communication	1/5 relevant criteria

Abbreviations used: NR = not reported